Communicating in Professions and Organizations

Series editor
Jonathan Crichton
University of South Australia
Adelaide, SA, Australia

This ground-breaking series is edited by Jonathan Crichton, Senior Lecturer in Applied Linguistics at the University of South Australia. It provides a venue for research on issues of language and communication that matter to professionals, their clients and stakeholders. Books in the series explore the relevance and real world impact of communication research in professional practice and forge reciprocal links between researchers in applied linguistics/discourse analysis and practitioners from numerous professions, including healthcare, education, business and trade, law, media, science and technology.

Central to this agenda, the series responds to contemporary challenges to professional practice that are bringing issues of language and communication to the fore. These include:

- The growing importance of communication as a form of professional expertise that needs to be made visible and developed as a resource for the professionals
- Political, economic, technological and social changes that are transforming communicative practices in professions and organisations
- Increasing mobility and diversity (geographical, technological, cultural, linguistic) of organisations, professionals and clients

Books in the series combine up to date overviews of issues of language and communication relevant to the particular professional domain with original research that addresses these issues at relevant sites. The authors also explore the practical implications of this research for the professions/ organisations in question.

We are actively commissioning projects for this series and welcome proposals from authors whose experience combines linguistic and professional expertise, from those who have long-standing knowledge of the professional and organisational settings in which their books are located and joint editing/authorship by language researchers and professional practitioners.

The series is designed for both academic and professional readers, for scholars and students in Applied Linguistics, Communication Studies and related fields, and for members of the professions and organisations whose practice is the focus of the series.

More information about this series at
http://www.palgrave.com/series/14904

Staci Defibaugh

Nurse Practitioners and the Performance of Professional Competency

Accomplishing Patient-centered Care

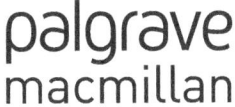

Staci Defibaugh
English
Old Dominion University
Norfolk, VA, USA

Communicating in Professions and Organizations
ISBN 978-3-319-68353-9   ISBN 978-3-319-68354-6 (eBook)
DOI 10.1007/978-3-319-68354-6

Library of Congress Control Number: 2017955941

© The Editor(s) (if applicable) and The Author(s) 2018, corrected publication [February/2018]
This work is subject to copyright. All rights are solely and exclusively licensed by the Publisher, whether the whole or part of the material is concerned, specifically the rights of translation, reprinting, reuse of illustrations, recitation, broadcasting, reproduction on microfilms or in any other physical way, and transmission or information storage and retrieval, electronic adaptation, computer software, or by similar or dissimilar methodology now known or hereafter developed.
The use of general descriptive names, registered names, trademarks, service marks, etc. in this publication does not imply, even in the absence of a specific statement, that such names are exempt from the relevant protective laws and regulations and therefore free for general use.
The publisher, the authors and the editors are safe to assume that the advice and information in this book are believed to be true and accurate at the date of publication. Neither the publisher nor the authors or the editors give a warranty, express or implied, with respect to the material contained herein or for any errors or omissions that may have been made. The publisher remains neutral with regard to jurisdictional claims in published maps and institutional affiliations.

Cover illustration: © John Rawsterne/patternhead.com

Printed on acid-free paper

This Palgrave Macmillan imprint is published by Springer Nature
The registered company is Springer International Publishing AG
The registered company address is: Gewerbestrasse 11, 6330 Cham, Switzerland

The original version of this book was revised.
An erratum to this book can be found at
https://doi.org/10.1007/978-3-319-68354-6_7

Preface

The field of medical discourse research has long focused on interactional patterns of doctor–patient communication. Research in this subfield has provided a wealth of knowledge on how the medical visit is structured and how interactional practices allow providers to control the visit and reproduce the institutional asymmetry, and even has begun to make headway in improving medical care through intervention studies as well as efforts of linguistic and discourse analytic researchers to make their research available and accessible to a wide variety of audiences. Despite these accomplishments, one of the shortcomings of discourse-based research of healthcare visits is that the primary focus of study is medical doctors (MDs), minimizing the role that other provider types play in health care. In the United States, primary medical care is often delivered not by MDs, but by nurse practitioners (NPs) and physician assistants (PAs), both of which have been noticeably absent in the discourse analytic research of medical visits. One of the main purposes of this book, then, is to add to our collective understanding of how medical care is delivered in the United States by focusing on the interactional practices of NPs. In doing so, my hope is to contribute to the already existing body of research on doctor–patient interactions and encourage others to continue this line of research on NPs as well as other providers who may draw on different resources in their talk with patients than what has been previously noted. By examining the practices of other provider types such as NPs, we can gain a more nuanced and more accurate understanding of healthcare discourse as it is delivered today.

I want to be clear that this book is not meant to be a comparison of the interactional practices of NPs and MDs. This would be an overreach of the data and an unfair comparison since there are many factors that contribute to how talk is carried out in medical visits. For example, in Chap. 2, I discuss some of the organizational responsibilities of the NPs in this study and how these responsibilities influence their interactions with patients. In this way, an equitable comparison could come only from the examination of MDs and NPs both working within the same organization. Rather than seeking to create a comparison, my intention is to provide an account of how NPs interact with patients in both inpatient and outpatient settings. Although the number of NPs in this study is relatively small, they represent three different clinical settings: inpatient care, outpatient care in a specialty clinic, and outpatient primary care. Future work may draw on the features discussed in this book for a comparison study, but at present, that is beyond the scope of this work.

The second main contribution of this book is to consider interactional practices as part of what it means to perform or enact a professional identity and to connect this to research outside of linguistics and discourse analytic studies. In order to do this, I examined four major themes that emerged in the data and connect those to the idea of professional competency as defined by health communication researchers and medical accreditation boards. Health communication researchers have long focused on what 'good' healthcare delivery looks like through the focus on patient satisfaction surveys and analysis of patient outcomes. However, what this may look like in practice is often outside the scope of these studies. Therefore, I hope to build connections, albeit preliminary, between the findings of health communication scholars and that of linguistic research, noting the ways in which particular aspects of healthcare delivery are performed on a turn-by-turn basis through a close textual analysis. Again, a caveat seems to be in order. By connecting this discourse analytic study of NP–patient interactions to the concept of professional competency, it is neither my goal nor within my capacity as a linguist to evaluate the work that the NPs in this study do. In discussing the data in terms of the performance of professional competency, I am not taking an evaluative stance; my goal is simply to draw larger connections to research outside of linguistics in order to better understand the interactional practices of NPs and to view them within the larger context of how medical care is conceptualized and understood across research and clinical disciplines.

Acknowledgments

Although there are many people who have provided tremendous support and encouragement for me throughout the process of writing this book, I absolutely could not have completed the work without the participation of the NPs and patients. I am forever indebted to the NPs for their willingness to allow me into their workspaces and for the patients for allowing me to record the often very private and personal space of their healthcare visit. This takes a great deal of trust, and I hope that I have not let them down in any way.

CONTENTS

1 Introduction   1

2 Frontstage/Backstage: Attending to Organizational Responsibilities   27

3 Need to Know: Patient Education and Epistemic Responsibility   53

4 Treading Lightly: Indirect Speech in Medical Directives   79

5 Caring as Competent: Small Talk in Medical Visits   101

6 Conclusion   121

Erratum   E1

Index   131

LIST OF TRANSCRIPTION CONVENTIONS

[	overlapping speech
=	latching, or no gap between utterances
-	cut-off speech
?	rising intonation phrase finally
↑	rising intonation word initially
,	continuing intonation
.	falling intonation
:	elongated sound
CAPS	loud speech
> <	fast speech
°okay°	quiet speech
underline	marked stress
###	unintelligible speech
(.)	pauses, marked with either the length in seconds or as (.) when less than 0.5 sec
Bold	focus of analysis

CHAPTER 1

Introduction

Abstract Healthcare visits with nurse practitioners (NPs) are becoming more common in the United States. Despite their growing numbers, we know little about NPs' interactional practices. This book addresses this gap in the literature by providing a discourse analytic account of NP–patient interactions. In this introductory chapter, prior research on NPs' effectiveness as healthcare providers lays the groundwork for the analytical chapters which follow. The book considers how NPs' interactional practices align with the concept of professional 'competency'; therefore, a discussion of how 'competency' is defined in terms of effective communication and its link to positive health outcomes and patient satisfaction is discussed. The chapter concludes with a discussion of the research context and a brief description of the remaining chapters.

Keywords Nurse practitioners • Patient satisfaction • Health outcomes • Competency • Patient-centered care

1 INTRODUCTION

The primary goal of this book is to present an analysis of the interactional practices of nurse practitioners (NPs) during medical visits with patients. The approach I take, which is to examine the particular linguistic choices that NPs employ, addresses an important gap in the research as the majority of discourse-based studies of medical interactions have focused almost exclusively on medical doctors (MDs). However, as healthcare delivery in the United States continues to shift, NPs are becoming more prominent figures in health care. Therefore, understanding their interactional practices and situating those practices within the context of their educational and training background as well as the prior research on their effectiveness are essential. Not only are NP–patient visits becoming the norm in the United States, because of their educational background in nursing and their patient-centered, holistic approach, NPs represent a new power dynamic (Defibaugh, 2014a) and one that must be explored more fully in order to present an accurate portrait of provider–patient visits in the United States.

This introductory chapter provides a theoretical and empirical grounding for the analytic chapters that follow. As such, I provide background on NPs as a provider type, including information on their educational background and training, the role that they play in US health care, and the existing research on NPs' effectiveness in terms of patient satisfaction and health outcomes. I also operationalize the concept of 'professional competency' by drawing on prior research in health communication and the way that competencies are defined by various medical accreditation boards. The chapter concludes with a description of the data that will be drawn on in subsequent chapters, including descriptions of the clinical sites and background information on the NPs that participated in the study.

2 Nurse Practitioners: A Growing Presence in US Health Care

NPs are a subgroup of Advanced Practice Registered Nurses (APRN), who work in a variety of settings and specialties, including primary care, emergency, oncology, and women's health. NPs typically hold either an MS in Nursing (MSN) or Doctor of Nursing Practice (DNP) degree, which requires an additional two to four years of full-time education beyond the four-year RN degree (Explore Health Careers, 2013) as well as 500–700 supervised clinical hours (Iglehart, 2013). NPs are licensed by the individual states in which they practice and must pass a national certification exam (AANP, 2017). Similar to medical doctors (MDs), NPs may specialize in their degree programs and can seek employment in a variety of inpatient and outpatient settings. Reports indicate that approximately 93–94% of NPs are female (US Department of Health and Human Services, 2014; Skilman, Kaplan, Fordyce, McMenamin, & Doescher, 2012).

The number of nurse practitioners practicing in the United States has been steadily increasing over the past two decades. The American Association of Nurse Practitioners (AANP) states that there were over 220,000 licensed NPs in the United States as of 2016, with numbers projected to increase to 244,000 by 2025 (AANP, 2017). The steady increase reflects the greater presence that NPs have in health care in the United States. One trend in health care that may partially account for the growing number of NPs is the current shortage of primary care physicians, particularly felt in rural areas and inner cities where physicians are less likely to practice (Goodell, Dower, & O'Neil, 2011). With only about 30% of all US physicians practicing in primary care, an amount totaling approximately 200,000 primary care physicians (National Center for Health Care Statistics, 2011), many areas are underserved. Bodenheimer and Pham (2010) report that many people live in areas where the ratio of patients to primary care providers is approximately 2000 to 1. The AANP statistics note that only 14.5% of physicians entered a primary care residency in 2016, again highlighting the continuously low numbers of MDs practicing in primary care and the increased need for alternative providers such as NPs to fill this gap. Auerbach et al. (2013) project that by 2025, physicians will represent only about 60% of all primary care providers—a drop of 11% from where they were in 2013, when the data were reported. They suggest that the ratio of MDs to NPs in primary care will be 2:1, respectively (Auerbach et al., 2013). In the Veterans Affairs (VA) system, NPs currently make up approximately 20% of all primary care visits and fulfill similar roles as MDs (Morgan, Abbott, McNeil, & Fisher, 2012).

As NPs are taking a more prominent role in healthcare delivery in the United States, many states are also changing regulations, allowing for greater NP autonomy (Gadbois, Miller, Tyler, & Intrator, 2015). As of 2016, NPs have prescriptive privileges in all 50 states and the District of Columbia, and according to the AANP, 95.8% of practicing NPs prescribe medications. Twenty-six states in the United States allow NPs to practice autonomously. The research collected for this book was conducted in Indiana and Illinois. In these two states, NPs may be designated as primary care providers (PCPs); at the time of data collection, both Illinois and Indiana required what is known as 'physician oversight' (Barton

Associates, 2017), a somewhat vague term that refers to some level of supervision by or coordination with an MD. What this means in practice varies and is often dependent on the organization and/or physician (personal communication). Gadbois et al. (2015) similarly note that while some states make explicit the regulations for practice of NPs and physician assistants (PAs), many states use vague language making it difficult to determine what the scope of practice for NPs and PAs actually is. In the VA system, the site of the outpatient visits included in this book, NPs see patients independently but have a coordinating physician who reviews their charts biweekly and provides guidance when questions arise. The NP in this study working at a community hospital also sees patients independently but works with a team of physicians, none of which 'oversee' her practice but coordinate care with her.

The shift in the make-up of health care, particularly in primary care, has led to an increased presence of NPs and an expansion of their scope of practice in many states. As health care continues to change in the United States from a primarily doctor-centered culture to one that includes other provider types such as NPs or PAs, nurse practitioner–patient interactions are an important and under-researched area of study, which can provide insight into the new medical model of healthcare delivery, which takes a more holistic and patient-centered perspective. As the following section notes, NPs have a presence in US health care for decades, and their training and focus on patient-centered care has already been well documented in the literature; however, the fine-grained linguistic analysis of these interactions is an area that deserves more attention as it can provide a more comprehensive understanding of the language used in healthcare delivery in the United States today.

3 Nurse Practitioners: Prior Research

3.1 Nurse Practitioner–Patient Interactions

Although discourse and conversation analysts have been studying doctor–patient interactions since the 1970s, very little research has focused on nurse practitioners. While Sally Candlin's (c.f. 2000, 2010) work on nurse–patient interactions comes the closest to providing a systematic account of how the occupation of nursing is constructed in medical interactions, her research focuses on registered nurses (RNs), rather than NPs, a role with a very different position within the medical community and a different context for interaction. In my own work on nurse practitioner–patient visits, I have noted the ways in which NPs seek to create solidarity with patients by minimizing the inherent asymmetry of the medical visits through the use of indirect speech (Defibaugh, 2014b) and aligning with patients' narrative experiences (Defibaugh, 2014a); however, these two studies alone do not provide the type of comprehensive account of NP–patient interactions that this book contributes.

Two earlier discourse-based studies offered a comparison of NPs with other providers (Drass, 1988; Fisher, 1991). Fisher analyzes two similar medical visits, one involving a doctor and the other an NP. In this comparison, she notes that the NP in the study delves into the patient's social life, focusing on nonmedical causes of her fatigue, while the MD restricts his questions to biomedical concerns, leaving issues in the realm of the social or psychological out of the medical interview. Drass (1988), similarly, compares an NP with two PAs working in the same clinic. He notes that the NP is more attentive to the voice of the lifeworld (Mishler, 1984) and engages in more nonrestrictive, open-ended questions than the PAs. In his discussion of how the different providers discuss treatment options, he notes that the NP "goes beyond these topics [the presenting problem] and addresses important lifeworld concerns of her patients" (Drass, 1988, p. 179). Although important for providing micro-level analyses of NP–patient visits, neither of these studies focuses exclusively on the interactional practices of NPs; instead, they both offer a comparison which places NPs in a position of the 'other.' This is most clearly the case in Fisher's comparison with a doctor, the unmarked provider type in primary care visits and in medical discourse research, but even in Drass' study, his comparison of NPs and PAs positions NPs as the alternative from PAs who follow a similar trajectory as doctors and take a "traditional medical perspective" (165).

Although outside the field of discourse analysis, and therefore lacking linguistic analysis, per se, Seale, Anderson, and Kinnersley (2005) also offer a comparison study of interactional practices of NPs and MDs, this time involving 12 interactions in total. Their study takes a more quantitative approach, indicating statistically significant differences in the amount of time and the number of options that NPs discuss during the treatment and diagnosis phase. They found that NPs' discussion of treatment options was significantly longer than that of doctors, with specific focus on how the treatment would work along with a discussion of side effects. They also noted that NPs recommended a greater number of treatment options to their patients. This study is revealing in its comparison of MDs and NPs, noting aspects of healthcare communication that differ for NP, but again, does not necessarily address, with any specificity, the ways in which NPs interact with patients. This book adds to this and the previously mentioned research by addressing ways in which NPs exhibit their professional competency by examining interactional data from both inpatient and outpatient settings by utilizing discourse analytic methods.

3.2 Nurse Practitioners, Patient Satisfaction, and Positive Health Outcomes

Beyond the research on communication practices, there is a great deal of research related to patient satisfaction and positive health outcomes for patients who seek medical care from a nurse practitioner.

Within the research on patient satisfaction, studies indicate that NPs have either equal or better patient satisfaction ratings than MDs or PAs. Some studies have indicated similar satisfaction rates of NPs and MDs (Dierick-van Daele, Metsemakers, Derckx, Spreeuwenberg, & Vrijhoef, 2009; Lenz, Mundinger, Kane, Hopkins, & Lin, 2004; Levine, Morlock, Mushlin, Shapiro, & Malitz, 1976; Merenstein, Wolfe, & Barker, 1974), highlighting the comparable quality of care delivered by NPs, based on post-visit surveys with patients. Other studies show higher satisfaction rates for NPs (Horrocks, Anderson, & Salisbury, 2002; Newhouse et al., 2011; Seale et al., 2005). Patients often report being more responsive to NPs' communication style and claim they would more likely adhere to the plan of treatment (Baratt, 2005; Charlton, Dearing, Berry, & Johnson, 2008). Budzi, Lurie, Singh, and Hooker (2010) surveyed patients seen by NPs, PAs, and MDs at VA medical centers. Overall, survey respondents were more satisfied with the care they received from NPs than PAs and MDs, and claimed that they preferred to see an NP rather than a PA or a physician. Some of the reasons for the preference were cited as NPs' focus on disease prevention, health education, and a higher level of attentiveness during the medical visit.

One commonly held belief about NPs and a reason sometimes given for their higher satisfaction ratings is that NPs have more time with patients. In a study conducted in the Netherlands, researchers noted that it was the case that the NPs spent more time with patients than their MD counterparts (Dierick-van Daele et al., 2009); however, other research indicates no statistically significant difference (Guzik, Menzel, Fitzpatrick,

& McNulty, 2009). For the NPs who participated in this study, they are not given more time by their organization. Within the VA system, NPs are treated the same as MDs or PAs and are scheduled for 30-minute visits for primary care or chronic care follow-up visits. Whether NPs utilize more of that 30-minute time frame compared to other providers working in the same setting cannot be determined as this research focuses solely on NPs and no data were collected on other providers working in the clinic. 'June,' who works in a community hospital, directs her practice in similar ways as the MDs she works with, seeing as many patients as she effectively can in any given work day; again, no data were collected with other providers working in this setting, so no actual comparison can be. The AANP reports that 60% of NPs see three or more patients per hour (AANP, 2017), which although not conclusive of the claim that they have an equal amount of time with patients does illustrate the fact that NPs face similar time demands in their practice as other medical providers.

In addition to the research on patient satisfaction, many studies indicate comparable or better health outcomes by patients who see an NP. For example, Ohman-Strikland and colleagues (2008) report that family practice offices that employed NPs provided better care for patients with diabetes than offices with MDs alone or MDs and PAs. Although intriguing, the specific role of the NP in this difference is not the focus of the study and, therefore, is not discussed in the article, leaving it unclear exactly what influence the NPs may have had on diabetes patients in this study. In a meta-analysis of 37 journal articles, researchers found that NPs were comparable to MDs on patient outcomes, including (1) patient satisfaction, (2) number of emergency department visits and hospitalizations following treatment, (3) blood glucose and blood pressure levels, and (4) mortality rates (Stanik-Hutt et al., 2013). Additionally, they found that patients who were cared for by an NP had better cholesterol levels than those who received care from an MD (also reported in Lenz et al., 2004). Patients seeing an NP for weight loss intervention in the Netherlands also had better health outcomes, with a higher percentage of weight loss than those who visited an MD (ter Bogt et al., 2009). The results of these studies indicate that the quality of care provided by NPs is comparable to that of MDs and, in some cases, may even be better, illustrating the importance of NPs in the healthcare landscape of the United States and further supporting the need to understand the linguistic mechanisms that may contribute to these positive health outcomes.

One reason for the positive outcomes and satisfaction results may be attributed to the patient-centered approach of NPs. Although not explicitly defined as such, the patient-centered approach has been recognized as the hallmark of NP practice (Cunningham, 2004). Patient-centered care, which takes an alternative approach to older, more traditional, physician-centered health care, has increased in popularity since the 1970s (Robinson, Callister, Berry, & Dearing, 2008). Robinson and colleagues cite the Institute of Medicine's definition of patient-centered care as "a partnership among practitioners, patients, and their families (when appropriate) to ensure that decisions respect patient's wants, needs, and preferences and that patients have the education and support they need to make decisions and participate in their own care" (cited in Robinson et al., 2008). Stewart and colleagues offer a similar definition that involves six components including approaching care from a holistic perspective, considering the patient's experiences with his/her illness, a focus on education and wellness, and working to enhance the provider–patient relationship. These values are highlighted in the AANP's description of their 'unique approach' to health care:

> What sets NPs apart from other health care providers is their unique emphasis on the health and well-being of the whole person. With a focus on health promotion, disease prevention, and health education and counseling, NPs guide patients in making smarter health and lifestyle choices, which in turn can lower patients' out-of-pocket costs. (AANP, 2017)

The focus on holistic health and education, as AANP promotes, correlates well with the definition of patient-centered care (Stewart et al., 2000), as both highlight treating the whole person, rather than the illness, and greater concern for long-term health through focus on disease preventions and lifestyle changes.

As this section has indicated, NPs have been proven to be effective healthcare providers both in the United States and in Europe, where many of the studies cited above were conducted. What is interesting about this body of research is that NPs have high satisfaction rates and high patient outcomes despite their lower level of social status in the United States compared to MDs. They are often referred to by the term 'mid-level' provider, suggesting that they reside in an intermediary position between MDs and RNs, a term that many NPs actively resist because of the connotation that they provide a lower level of care or lower quality of care than their physician counterparts despite performing many of the same roles. NPs have also come up against resistance in their push for autonomy, often by MDs who argue that NPs do not have the same level of knowledge or training as MDs (Jauhar, 2014). There is also the social difference in that NPs do not have a title equivalent to MDs, who are referred to by the title 'doctor' + last name; NPs often use their first name only. Despite all of this, the research indicates that NPs provide equally high-quality health care. Therefore, one of the goals of this book is to examine the particular linguistic practices that NPs employ in their work and attempt to connect these to the widely recognized and agreed-upon understanding of what effective healthcare delivery looks like. To be clear, it is not the goal of this book to define what effective communication in healthcare settings is. This has already been noted by other scholars and incorporated into medical accreditation requirements of 'core competencies' (see next section). Instead, my goal is to examine what some of these aspects of 'competency' look like in practice for the NPs in this study. For example, rather than claiming that patient education is important in healthcare delivery, I argue that patient education may involve prioritizing certain information even if that means ignoring a patient's immediate concern (Chap. 3). Similarly, it is not my position to state that creating rapport between provider and patient is important; instead, I illustrate how rapport may be constructed through engaging in small talk at various points in the visit (Chap. 5) or to suggest that negotiation of treatment, at least in some circumstances, may take the form of using indirectness to give medical advice (Chap. 4). With that focus in mind, I now turn to prior research and the medical community's assessment of what quality healthcare delivery entails or what I term 'professional competency.'

4 What Is Professional Competency?

Competency, for the purposes of this book, is defined as the delivery of effective health care. In medical care, competency is often equated with technical skills (Callahan, 1984); however, Kak, Burkhalter, and Cooper (2001) also include the following in their description of medical competencies: acting in 'the helping role' and 'the teaching-coaching role,' skills in administering therapeutic interventions, and job-related competencies such as 'organizational and work-role competencies,' all of which fall outside the realm of purely technical skills. One study that examined patients' perceptions of medical competency notes that while technical skills are valued more in surgical wards, both technical and interpersonal skills are considered equally valuable by patients in other settings, such as primary care (Murakami, Imanaka, Kobuse, Lee, & Goto, 2010). For the most part, research that addresses effective healthcare delivery relies on measures of patient satisfaction and improved health outcomes, both of which are discussed below.

4.1 Competency and Patient Satisfaction

Patient satisfaction, which can be understood as "a measure of quality from the patient's perspective" (Guzik et al., 2009, p. 192), is significant for two reasons. First, health care in the United States is largely a consumer-driven industry in which it is important for patients to be satisfied with the care they receive (Vuori, 1991). Second, and more importantly, higher satisfaction ratings are aligned with better patient outcomes. That is, if patients are more satisfied with their visit and their provider, then they will be more likely to adhere to the treatment plan.

Patient satisfaction may be based on many factors, including the actual diagnosis or length of time they must wait to see a provider. However, patients overwhelmingly cite communication as an important, if not *the most* important, factor in their impressions of the visit (Ben-Sira, 1982; Oetzel et al., 2015; Roberts & Aruguete, 2000). Studies suggest that provider interaction is a "key correlate for patient satisfaction" (Oetzel et al., 2015, p. 974). Marcinowicz, Chlabicz, and Grebowski (2009) surveyed 36 patients from nine family practice offices and found that they rated interaction with their provider as the most important aspect of satisfaction. They note that 40% of the survey responses referenced aspects of communication, while only 12.9% referred to the providers' medical skills. Buller and Buller (1987) cite a positive correlation between providers' affective behavior and patient satisfaction. In a study by Kliems and Witt (2011), patients rated providers' willingness to take the "time to listen" as a prominent characteristic in evaluating the quality of health care. Heritage and Robinson (2006), similarly, point out that physicians' use of open-ended opening questions at the beginning of the visit led to higher satisfaction rates, which they posit may be more about the opportunities of explanation of symptoms and expression of concerns afforded to patients rather than the length of turn that is given to them.

The research linking patient satisfaction and adherence to treatment also highlights the role of effective communication. Zolnierek and

DiMatteo's (2009) meta-analysis of 127 studies notes a statistically significant correlation between provider communication and patient adherence. They report that patients are 19% less likely to adhere to the prescribed treatment when the communication is poor. Hayes (2007) reports on surveys conducted with 103 patients who received care from one of eight NPs working in a managed care setting. She surveyed patients on their satisfaction with the visit and their provider, their ability to recall the treatment plan, and their claim of likelihood to adhere to the treatment plan. Quantitatively, she noted correlations between patients' overall satisfaction and the likeliness for adherence. Qualitative results reported in the study include patients' reasons for their claims of adherence, including reference to personal trust, a belief that the NP has his/her best interest in mind, and professional confidence in the NP as an expert. As these studies illustrate, effective communication and overall positive rapport with the provider are integral in patients' satisfaction ratings.

4.2 Competency and Positive Health Outcomes

Beyond ratings of patient satisfaction, research suggests that positive communication is associated with effective healthcare delivery, as it relates to better health outcomes. In a study involving individuals with gastroesophageal reflux disease (GERD), participants cited failures in communication between themselves and their providers as well as interaction among providers as the greatest reasons for failure (Farup et al., 2011). The authors define communication failures as patients receiving insufficient information about the disease or treatment alternatives or doctors not recognizing the severity of symptoms presented by the patients. Studies also indicate that patients' management of diabetes is directly affected by their perception of their providers' ability to communicate effectively (Ciechanowski, Katon, Russo, & Walker, 2001; Parchman, Flannagan, Ferrer, & Matamoras, 2009). Both Ciechanowski et al. (2001) and Parchman et al. (2009) examined patients' A1C values (an empirical assessment of blood sugar levels over a three-to-four-month period) and compared these with either patients' evaluations of poor communication (Ciechanowski et al., 2001) or the researchers' own assessments of communication based on evaluation of the medical visits (Parchman et al., 2009). Parchman and colleagues noted that higher levels of communicative competence (assessed in terms of the following seven factors: rapport-building, information management, agenda setting, active listening, addressing feelings, reaching common ground and overall competence) by the physician were associated with better diabetes management by patients. Cierchanowksi and colleagues, similarly, found a correlation between positive evaluations of provider–patient communication with lower A1C levels, or better diabetes management.

4.3 Communication, Competency, and Medical Accreditation Boards

Not only does the research show that communication is an integral part of what it means to be a competent and effective provider, medical accreditation boards also highlight the role of communication in how they define competency. The National Organization of Nurse Practitioner Faculties (NONPF), an organization created to implement standards for nurse practitioner education programs as well as benchmarks for successful completion of graduate programs in nursing, place a higher value on demonstration of achievement of the core competencies than the number of clinical hours performed as part of their educational program (NONPF, 2017). The NONPF divides the core competencies into nine categories: scientific foundation, leadership, quality, practice inquiry, technology information and literacy, policy, health delivery system, ethics, and independent practice. Although none of these competencies solely address communication or the patient-centered approach per se, there is evidence of these in almost every competency. For example, in both the 'scientific foundation' and 'technology and information literacy' competencies, reference is made to 'translating' research and scientific information to patients based on their needs. In the section entitled 'health delivery system,' they include the utilization of communication skills involved in "negotiating, consensus-building and partnering" (2017: 4); the independent practices section makes reference to the need for NPs to provide "the full spectrum of health care services including health promotion, disease prevention, health protection, anticipatory guidance, counseling, disease management, palliative and end of life care" (2017: 4) all of which are dependent on effective communication. Within this section, NONPF also includes a section that specifically addresses patient-centered care, which include the following four subcategories:

(a) Works to establish a relationship with the patient, characterized by mutual respect, empathy, and collaboration.
(b) Creates a climate of patient-centered care to include confidentiality, privacy, comfort, emotional support, mutual trust, and respect.
(c) Incorporates the patient's cultural and spiritual preferences, values, and beliefs into health care.
(d) Preserves the patient's control over decision making by negotiating a mutually acceptable plan of care.

Note that both (a) and (b) specifically address ways in which NPs should create relationships with patients, including through the show of empathy (a) and creating an atmosphere of comfort and support (b), features they consider both part of the patient-centered approach as well as important factors for the successful delivery of medical care. The focus of (c), although not immediately relevant to the data presented in this book, does highlight the importance of the holistic approach to patients, viewing them as discreet, yet complex individuals whose identities extend beyond their illness or their immediate, institutional identity of 'patient.' Finally, (d) emphasizes the need for NPs to work with patients, providing them options and working in tandem rather than in a purely authoritarian position. It is clear from the NONPF's competencies that communication and patient-centeredness are important factors in what they consider to be effective medical training for NPs.

The inclusion of similar features in accreditation boards for other medical providers—namely, MDs—highlights the fact that these features associated with patient-centered care and effective communication are part of what it means to be a competent medical doctor as well. The Accreditation Council for Graduate Medical Education (ACGME), which provides accreditation for residency and fellowship programs at medical institutions in the United States, also provides a comprehensive list of competencies with which they use to evaluate residency programs. Their list of competencies is somewhat different but includes 'interpersonal and communication skills' as one of the six main categories. This category specifies that residents "must demonstrate interpersonal and communication skills that result in the effective exchange of information and collaboration with patients, their families, and health professionals" (ACGME, 2016, p. 11). Similarly, the American Board of Medical Specialties (ABMS), a board that oversees ongoing accreditation or medical specialists, also includes "interpersonal and communication skills" as one of their six competencies. They specify this competency as including use of "effective listening skills with non-verbal and verbal communication" (2017, para. 6).

It is important to note that NPs are not assessed by any of these boards and that the purpose of including them is not to suggest that the interactional practices of NPs be judged by these standards. I include them to illustrate that there is consensus in the research community as well as the medical community that effective communication is important to the delivery of quality health care. Although the focus of this book is on NPs and their performance of professional competency, what is understood as competent by the research and medical governing bodies could be applied to other provider types as well. Indeed, although there is consensus on what competency is, there is little research that addresses what these competencies looks like in terms of specific interactional practices and linguistic choices.

As this chapter has shown so far, communication is an integral part of the delivery of quality health care. Also, it has been shown that NPs are able to deliver quality health care to patients, as evidenced by their high patient satisfaction ratings and the positive health outcomes that their patients are able to achieve. This book contributes to the research by delving deeper into what those communicative practices are using as discourse analytic methods and examining interactions between nurse practitioners and patients. The remainder of this chapter provides contextual information for the data presented in the book and a description of the chapters.

5 DATA FOR THE BOOK

The data presented in this book are based on research collected with five NPs working in three different settings. The earlier research was conducted with 'June,' who works in a nonprofit community hospital located in a mid-sized city in the Midwestern region of the United States. The primary data source was audio recordings of visits between June and her patients. Because of the inpatient setting where patients primarily had large private rooms, I was present during these interactions, positioning myself outside of the line of sight of June and the patient. As a supporting data source, extensive field notes were collected with June as she made her rounds with patients and consulted the patients' electronic records both before and after each visit. June would often share with me, prior to the visit, what her goals were when meeting with each patient, based on what she had read in the medical records. Because of this, and the fact that I was able to be present during the visits, I have greater knowledge of the context of these visits compared to those collected in the other settings.

A second data collection took place at two different VA locations[1] also located in the Midwest. The first site was a cardiac care clinic located within a large, regional hospital located in an urban, downtown setting. The NP working in this location is 'Julie,' whose primary role in this clinic was to provide ongoing care for patients prior to having cardiac surgery. The second site was a VA outpatient clinic, where I collected data with three NPs: 'Karen,' 'Laura,' and 'Sarah.' For both of these sites, the primary data collection was audio recordings of medical visits. However, due to the small size of the medical rooms, I felt that my presence would be distracting for both the NPs and the patients and, therefore, I was not present during the visits. In addition to the audio recordings, I conducted structured interviews with patients after each visit as well as semi-structured interviews with the NPs, all of which were audio-recorded. When appropriate, data gleaned from these sources will be used to support the analysis of the medical visits, but they are not the primary analytic focus of this book.

More detailed information on the NPs in this study and the clinical settings is provided below. Focus is placed mainly on the NPs, their training, and scope of individual practice. Brief descriptions of the clinical settings are included in each section as further contextualization for the data analysis chapters.

5.1   NPs in This Study

5.1.1   June

June works in a 320-bed community hospital located in a semi-urban city in the Midwest. The hospital serves both the city and the smaller, more rural towns in the area. She is the diabetes specialist on an internal medicine team working with approximately 20 other providers. She holds a master's degrees in nursing (MSN) and is designated as a Family Nurse Practitioner (FNP). Her role with patients is multifaceted, the main task being to set or adjust insulin dosages for patients, both while in the hospital and upon discharge. She also fulfills the role of diabetes educator by answering patients' questions, ensuring they understand what to do when they go home, and aiding in making certain that resources are available for patients, specifically in terms of access to medication, since many patients do not have insurance or the financial ability to pay for their insulin. She sees as many patients as she can in a day based on need (i.e. blood sugar readings), including initial and follow-up visits, many of which are arranged to discuss specific topics and to provide education to patients and their family members. She must balance spending as much time as needed with each patient and seeing as many people as she can. Therefore, the more time she spends with one may be taking her away from others. She may see some patients multiple times in one day (although more than twice is rare) and may see the same patient only once during any given hospitalization or many times, depending on the length of hospitalization and the perceived need for diabetes management. Because of this variability, an average number of patients per day is difficult to determine and may present an inaccurate picture of her practice. The average length of each medical visit that was recorded as part of this research is 15 minutes, but interactions range from just over two minutes to 45 minutes. The variation in length is somewhat typical for inpatient visits in which providers make their rounds with patients and are not constrained by a pre-set schedule of appointments as is typical in outpatient care.

5.1.2 Julie

Julie works in the cardiac clinic in a VA hospital in an urban downtown location. This hospital provides many services and often serves a diverse population in terms of race, ethnicity, and socio-economic status to former members of the US military. Julie balances her time between the cardiac clinic in the downtown hospital, a primary care clinic in a suburban location, as well as leading a weight-management support group (also at the main hospital). Data collected with Julie consisted of the cardiac clinic visits only. In this location, Julie's primary role was to conduct follow-up appointments to assess medication management for individuals who had previously undergone cardiac surgery. These patients were required, on a regular basis (often around 3–6 months), to get blood work taken and discuss the results with the NP, who would then make medication adjustments as necessary. Julie also assessed patients' current cardiac health, discussing exercise routines, dietary habits, and any signs for continuing cardiac problems. Julie started her career at the VA as an RN and also worked part-time in the private sector for approximately five years before getting her master's degree in nursing (MSN) to become an NP. She had worked as an NP for 17 years, all of which had been at the VA at the time of data collection.

5.1.3 Karen, Laura, and Sarah

Karen, Laura, and Sarah all work at a VA clinic located in a suburban area. The clinic is composed of smaller clinics (e.g. women's health, optometry, audiology) as well as an onsite pharmacy, phlebotomy lab, and radiology lab. All three NPs work in the men's health clinic with patients who are retired from the US military. Most of the patients that come to this clinic live in suburban areas and travel less than 30 miles for visits. Most of the patients, as reported by one NP, and supported by my observations, have private insurance and a private doctor, meaning that they see a primary care provider outside of the VA, and typically come to the VA for an annual checkup only. The benefits of being in the VA system are that patients can get more affordable prescriptions (and the convenience of mailed medications without additional paperwork) and access to affordable, sometimes free, tests and immunizations. However, for many of them, the VA is not close to their home and the desire to have access to a medical provider in their home town is appealing and worth the added expense of private/employer health insurance and/or Medicare. Visits in this clinic were scheduled in 30-minute intervals for all patients except for those seeking care at the VA for the first time; for these patients, a visit of 60 minutes was scheduled.

Of the three NPs at this location, Laura had the greatest amount of experience. She worked for 13 years as an RN, including time spent as a medic in the army. She was the only NP in this study who was also a military veteran herself. In addition to her 13 years as an RN, she also had 18 years of experience as a practicing NP at the time of the study, all of which were within the VA system. Karen had been practicing as an NP for 14 years at the time that the research was conducted. She first earned her associate's degree in nursing and then enrolled in an accelerated program to complete her MSN. Unlike many NPs, she did not practice as an RN before earning her master's degree nor did she have any experience working in any setting other than the VA. Sarah worked six years as an RN before and during graduate school. She had been practicing as an NP for 14 years: eight years in the private sector; six years at the VA. She explained that she preferred working in the VA because of the autonomy that NPs had, compared to the private sector. She also commented on the fact that within the

VA system, they got more time to spend with patients and were able to perform a true primary care role, which differed from her earlier experiences.

5.2 Transcription Information

The medical visits and interviews were all audio-recorded and transcribed following conventions outlined by Gail Jefferson (cited in Atkinson & Heritage, 2006) with noted features such as length and placement of pauses, simultaneous and overlapping speech, and prosodic features, including stress and intonation. All identifying information was changed, including pseudonyms for participants, other medical providers referenced in the interactions and names of cities, hospitals, and other identifying locations in order to maintain the anonymity of participants. All of the NPs in this study refer to patients by title and last name (e.g. Mr. Barnes), but use their first name when introducing themselves to patients. I have chosen to follow this naming practice in the way that I refer to the patients and the NPs both in the text and the transcripts to reflect their preferred forms of address.

6 Organization of the Book

One of the goals of this book is to examine the linguistic practices that NPs engage in throughout their interactions with patients. Much of the research on medical discourse starts from the perspective of the medical visit as involving a set of distinct transactional phases (i.e. history taking/ examination, diagnosis, etc.). Research often focuses on one aspect of the visit, for example, openings and problem presentation or the diagnostic phase of the visit. Rather than take this approach, I look at the different roles that NPs play within the visit, which often occur across different phases of the visit. For this reason, the book is organized thematically based on specific interactional practices rather than linearly and based on transactional phases. Chapters are designed to address specific aspects of the NPs' professional role and the ways in which they perform this role. The following paragraphs provide a brief description of the rest of the book and its organization.

Chapter 2 considers how NPs address their organizational responsibilities within the medical visit. Not often discussed in the medical discourse research, the ways in which these 'backstage' organizational responsibilities get enacted during the 'frontstage' of medical visits often influences the talk that occurs between provider and patient. In this chapter, I discuss two ways in which organizational responsibilities are referenced or enacted during the medical visit. First, in outpatient visits in the VA clinic, NPs must attend to patients' electronic medical records (EMRs) and must, more or less, follow the 'scripting' of these EMRs, which then dictates the talk during the visit. Second, I focus on the ways that June, working in an inpatient setting, makes explicit reference to the work that happens behind the scenes in the coordination of care for patients. Drawing the metaphor of 'frontstage/backstage' (Goffman, 1959), I argue that unlike many of Goffman's examples, the performance of medical competency involves revealing the backstage work rather than hiding it from patients.

Chapter 3 focuses on an important aspect of medical care: information sharing and patient education. Utilizing Stivers, Mondada, and Steensig's (2011) 'dimensions of knowledge,' I examine a number of ways in which NPs share knowledge with patients. One of the defining features of the NPs' approach, according to the AANP, is patient education. Not only must NPs decide what information patients need during a particular visit, they must also consider how best to convey that information. In this chapter, I argue that in order to provide education to patients, NPs must prioritize patients' need for certain information, or their 'epistemic primacy' (Stivers et al., 2011) over assessing prior knowledge. Additionally, I point out how addressing 'primacy' may include foregrounding some information while backgrounding other, less significant, information as well as how NPs may employ different registers (including using more or less medical jargon) to tailor the form of information based on patients' current knowledge.

Chapter 4 examines the ways in which medical advice and instructions are communicated to patients. This chapter complements the previous chapter's focus on education and moves toward what patients need to do when they leave the hospital or provider's office. In this chapter, I focus on the ways in which NPs use indirect speech when giving advice or instructions. One of the reasons posited for this use of indirectness is that advice often comes with criticism of past failures; indirectness allows the NPs to avoid directly criticizing patients and seemingly offer suggestions for healthy behaviors rather than handing down directives in an authoritarian manner. This provides room for negotiation with patients on some level as suggestions are open for interpretation while directives are not; it also reflects the patient-centered approach through the avoidance of the potential face threats associated with directives or commands.

Chapter 5 focuses even more on the enactment of the patient-centered approach by examining the ways is which rapport is constructed through small talk, or talk that is not directly related to the transactional goals of the visit. The chapter presents examples of small talk that occur at different places in the visit: the opening, the middle, and the closing, illustrating that NPs seek to create rapport with patients, which in turn can create a positive provider–patient relationship, a feature associated with the patient-centered approach. I argue that because small talk is often relatively short, it does not necessarily take away from the transactional work of the visit but can, in fact, contribute to it.

Chapter 6 brings together the data and discussion from the four analysis chapters and considers how each of these aspects of the NPs' role contributes to their performance of professional competency. I argue that the linguistic resources that NPs use in their enactment of a "competent" provider cannot be understood in a vacuum, that is, individual linguistic practices do not directly correlate with a specific aspect of the NPs' roles, but need to be understood holistically and collectively. I also discuss directions for future research.

7 Conclusion

The aim of this book is to illustrate some of the linguistic features associated with the NP's interactional style and position these features within the framework of the performance of professional competency. In doing so, I have selected four sites of linguistic analysis (referencing backstage work in the frontstage to highlight organizational responsibilities, adapting language use to provide appropriate patient education, mitigating medical advice through indirect speech, and engaging in small talk as a way of creating rapport), which will be the focus of the four analytical chapters that follow. In this chapter, I have provided contextual background for these analytical chapters. The description of prior research on NPs is by no means exhaustive but should provide sufficient background for the reader and justification for the focus on NPs both as an integral component of health care in the United States and as an under-researched provider in the field of medical discourse analysis as well as for the understanding of what is meant by professional competency and how this is accomplished through interaction.

Notes

1. The VA system provides health care for former US military personnel. It is one of the largest providers of health care in the United States (United States Department of Veterans Affairs, 2017).

References

Accreditation Council for Graduate Medical Education. (2016). *Core program requirements*. Retrieved July 17, 2017, from http://www.acgme.org/What-We-Do/Accreditation/Common-Program-Requirements

American Association of Nurse Practitioners. (2017). Retrieved May 24, 2017, from https://www.aanp.org/all-about-nps/what-is-an-np#license-and-practice-locations

American Board of Medical Specialties. (2017). Retrieved August 14, 2017, from http://www.abms.org/board-certification/a-trusted-credential/based-on-core-competencies

Atkinson, J. M., & Heritage, J. (2006). Jefferson's transcript notation. In A. Jaworski & N. Coupland (Eds.), *The discourse reader* (2nd ed., pp. 158–165).

Auerbach, D. I., Chen, P. G., Friedberg, M. W., Reid, R., Lau, C., Buerhaus, P. I., et al. (2013). Nurse-managed health centers and patient-centered medical homes could mitigate expected primary care physician shortage. *Health Affairs, 32*(11), 1933–1941.

Baratt, J. (2005). A case study of styles of patient self-presentation in the nurse practitioner primary health care consultation. *Primary Health Care Research and Development, 6*, 329–340.

Barton Associates. (2017). Retrieved July 19, 2017, from https://www.bartonassociates.com/locum-tenens-resources/nurse-practitioner-scope-of-practice-laws

Ben-Sira, Z. (1982). Stress potential and esotericity of health problems: The significance of the physician's affective behavior. *Medical Care, 20*, 414–424.

Bodenheimer, T., & Pham, H. H. (2010). Primary care: Current problems and proposed solutions. *Health Affairs, 29*, 799–805.

Budzi, D., Lurie, S., Singh, K., & Hooker, R. (2010). Veterans' perceptions of care by nurse practitioners, physician assistants, and physicians: A comparison from satisfaction surveys. *Journal of American Academy of Nurse Practice, 22*, 170–176.

Buller, J., & Buller, D. (1987). Physicians' communication styles and patient satisfaction. *Journal of Health and Social Behavior, 28*, 375–388.

Callahan, D. (1984). Competency in medical care. *Nebraska Law Review, 63*(4), 663.

Candlin, S. (2000). Ne dynamics in the nurse–patient relationship? In S. Sarangi & M. Coulthard (Eds.), *Discourse and social life*. London: Longman.

Candlin, S. (2010). 'We're just going to be talking about you...' Identifying deficits and achieving quality in nurse-patient discourse. In C. N. Candlin & J. Crichton (Eds.), *Discourses of deficit* (pp. 119–136).
Charlton, C., Dearing, K., Berry, J., & Johnson, M. J. (2008). Nurse practitioners' communication styles and their impact on patient outcomes: An integrated literature review. *Journal of the American Academy of Nurse Practitioners, 20*, 382–388.
Ciechanowski, P. S., Katon, W. J., Russo, J. E., & Walker, E. A. (2001). The patient-provider relationship: Attachment theory and adherence to treatment in diabetes. *American Journal of Psychiatry, 158*, 29–35.
Cunningham, R. S. (2004). Advanced nursing practice outcomes: A review of selected empirical literature. *Oncology Nursing Forum, 31*, 219–230.
Defibaugh, S. (2014a). Solidarity and alignment in nurse practitioner/patient interactions. *Discourse & Communication, 8*(3), 260–277.
Defibaugh, S. (2014b). Management of health or management of face: Indirectness in nurse practitioner-patient interactions. *Journal of Pragmatics, 67*, 61–71.
Dierick-van Daele, A. T., Metsemakers, J. F., Derckx, E. W., Spreeuwenberg, C., & Vrijhoef, H. J. (2009). Nurse practitioners substituting for general practitioners: Randomized controlled trial. *Journal of Advanced Nursing, 65*(2), 391–401.
Drass, K. A. (1988). Discourse and occupational perspective: A comparison of nurse practitioners and physician assistants. *Discourse Processes, 11*(2), 163–191.
Explore Health Careers. (2013). Retrieved November 23, 2013, from https://explorehealthcareers.org/career/nursing/nurse-practitioner
Farup, P., Blix, I., Forre, S., Johnsen, G., Lange, O., Johannessen, R., et al. (2011). What causes treatment failure – The patient, primary care, secondary care or inadequate interaction in the health services? *British Medical Journal Health Services Research, 11*, 1–6.
Fisher, S. (1991). A discourse of the social: Medical talk/power talk/oppositional talk? *Discourse & Society, 2*(2), 157–182.
Gadbois, E. A., Miller, E. A., Tyler, D., & Intrator, O. (2015). Trends in state regulation of nurse practitioners and physician assistants, 2001 to 2010. *Medical Care Research and Review, 72*(2), 200–219.
Goffman, E. (1959). *The presentation of self in everyday life*. Random House.
Goodell, S., Dower, C., & O'Neil, E. (2011). Primary care workforce in the United States. *Robert Wood Johnson Foundation Policy Brief, 22*. Retrieved from http://www.rwjf.org/content/dam/farm/reports/issue_briefs/2011/rwjf402104
Guzik, A., Menzel, N. N., Fitzpatrick, J., & McNulty, R. (2009). Patient satisfaction with NP and physician services in the occupational health setting. *American Association of Occupational Health Nurses Journal, 57*(5), 191–197.

Hayes, E. (2007). Nurse practitioners and managed care: Patient satisfaction and intention to adhere to nurse practitioner plan of care. *Journal of the American Academy of Nurse Practitioners, 19*, 418–426.

Heritage, J., & Robinson, J. (2006). The structure of patients' presenting concerns: Physicians' opening questions. *Health Communication, 19*(2), 89–102.

Horrocks, S., Anderson, E., & Salisbury, S. (2002). Systematic review of whether nurse practitioners working in primary care can provide equivalent care to doctors. *British Medical Journal, 324*, 819–823.

Iglehart, J. K. (2013). Expanding the role of advanced nurse practitioners: Risks and rewards. *The New England Journal of Medicine, 368*(20), 1935–1941.

Jauhar, S. (2014). Nurses are not doctors. *The New York Times*. Retrieved May 24, 2015, from http://www.nytimes.com/2014/04/30/opinion/nurses-are-not-doctors.html

Kak, N., Burkhalter, B., & Cooper, M. (2001). Measuring the competence of healthcare providers. *Operations Research Issue Paper, 2*(1). Bethesda, MD: Published for the U.S. Agency for International Development (USAID) by the Quality Assurance (QA) Project.

Kliems, H., & Witt, C. M. (2011). The good doctor: A qualitative study of German homeopathic physicians. *The Journal of Alternative and Complementary Medicine, 17*(3), 265–270.

Lenz, E. R., Mundinger, M. O., Kane, R. L., Hopkins, S. C., & Lin, S. X. (2004). Primary care outcomes in patients treated by nurse practitioners or physicians: Two-year follow-up. *Medical Care Research and Review, 61*, 332–351.

Levine, D. M., Morlock, L. L., Mushlin, A. I., Shapiro, S., & Malitz, F. E. (1976). The role of new health practitioners in a prepaid group practice: Provider differences in process and outcomes of medical care. *Medical Care, 14*(4), 326–347.

Marcinowicz, L., Chlabicz, S., & Grebowski, R. (2009). Patient satisfaction with healthcare provided by family doctors: Primary dimensions and an attempt at typology. *BMC Health Services Research, 9*, 63. https://doi.org/10.1186/1472-6963-9-63

Merenstein, J. H., Wolfe, H., & Barker, K. M. (1974). The use of nurse practitioners in a general practice. *Medical Care, 12*(5), 445–452.

Mishler, E. (1984). *The discourse of medicine: Dialectics of medical interviews.* Norwood, NJ: Ablex.

Morgan, P. A., Abbott, D. H., McNeil, R. B., & Fisher, D. A. (2012). Characteristics of primary care office visits to nurse practitioners, physician assistants and physicians in United States veterans health administration facilities, 2005 to 2010: A retrospective cross-sectional analysis. *Human Resources for Health, 10*(42), 1–8.

Murakami, G., Imanaka, Y., Kobuse, H., Lee, J., & Goto, E. (2010). Patient perceived priorities between technical skills and interpersonal skills: Their influence on correlates of patient satisfaction. *Journal of Evaluation in Clinical Practice, 16*, 560–568.

National Center for Health Statistics. (2011). *Health, United States, 2010: With special feature on death and dying*. Hyattsville, MD: National Center for Health Statistics.

National Organization for Nurse Practitioner Faculties. (2017). *Core competencies for nurse practitioners*. Retrieved May 17, 2017, from http://www.nonpf.org/?page=14

Newhouse, R. P., Stanik-Hutt, J., White, K. M., Johantgen, M., Bass, E. B., Zangaro, G., et al. (2011). Advanced practice nurse outcomes 1990–2008: A systematic review. *Nursing Economics, 29*, 230–251.

Oetzel, J., Wilcox, B., Avila, M., Hill, R., Archipoli, A., & Ginossar, T. (2015). Patient-provider interaction, patient satisfaction, and health outcomes: Testing explanatory models for people living with HIV/AIDS. *AIDS Care, 27*(8), 972–978.

Ohman-Strickland, P. A., Orzano, A. J., Solberg, L. I., Diciccio-Bloom, B., O'Malley, D., Tallia, A. F., et al. (2008). Quality of diabetes care in family medicine practices: Influence of nurse-practitioners and physician's assistants. *Annals of Family Medicine, 6*(1), 14–22.

Parchman, M. L., Flannagan, D., Ferrer, R. L., & Matamoras, M. (2009). Communication competence, self-care behaviors and glucose control in patients with type 2 diabetes. *Patient Education and Counseling, 77*, 55–59.

Roberts, C. A., & Aruguete, M. S. (2000). Task and socioemotional behaviors of physicians: A test of reciprocity and social interaction theories in analogue physician–patient encounters. *Social Science and Medicine, 50*, 309–315.

Robinson, J. H., Callister, L. C., Berry, J. A., & Dearing, K. A. (2008). Patient-centered care and adherence: Definitions and applications to improve outcomes. *Journal of the American Academy of Nurse Practitioners, 20*, 600–607.

Seale, C., Anderson, E., & Kinnersley, P. (2005). Treatment advice in primary care: A comparative study of nurse practitioners and general practitioners. *Issues and Innovations in Nursing Practice, 54*, 534–541.

Skilman, S. M., Kaplan, L., Fordyce, M. A., McMenamin, P., & Doescher, M. P. (2012). Understanding advanced practice registered nurse distribution in urban and rural areas of the United States using National Provider Identifier data. American Nurses Association Publication.

Stanik-Hutt, J., Newhouse, R. P., White, K. M., Johantgen, M., Bass, E. B., Zangaro, G., et al. (2013). The quality and effectiveness of care provided by nurse practitioners. *Journal of Nurse Practitioners, 9*(8), 492–499.

Stewart, M., Brown, J. B., Donner, D., McWhinney, I. R., Oates, J., Weston, W. W., et al. (2000). The impact of patient-centered care on outcomes. *The Journal of Family Practice, 49*(9), 796–804.

Stivers, T., Mondada, L., & Steensig, J. (2011). Knowledge, morality and affiliation in social interaction. In T. Stivers, L. Mondada, & J. Steensig (Eds.), *The morality of knowledge in conversation* (pp. 3–26). Cambridge: Cambridge University Press.

ter Bogt, N. C., Bemelmans, W. J., Beltman, F. W., Broer, J., Smit, A. J., & van der Meer, K. (2009). Preventing weight gain: One-year results of a randomized lifestyle intervention. *American Journal of Preventive Medicine, 37,* 270–277.

United States Department of Health and Human Services. (2014). *Health resources and services administration, national center for health workforce analysis. Highlights from the 2012 national sample survey of nurse practitioners.* Rockville, MD: U.S. Department of Health and Human Services.

United States Department of Veteran Affairs. (2017). Retrieved February 2, 2017, from https://www.va.gov/health

Vuori, H. (1991). Patient satisfaction—Does it matter? *International Journal for Quality in Health Care, 3*(3), 183–189.

Zolnierek, K. B. H., & DiMatteo, M. R. (2009). Physician communication and patient adherence to treatment: A meta-analysis. *Medical Care, 47*(8), 826–834.

CHAPTER 2

Frontstage/Backstage: Attending to Organizational Responsibilities

Abstract During healthcare visits, medical providers must attend to multiple agendas, including those of their patients and their organizations. A discussion of professional competency, then, must consider how nurse practitioners (NPs) attend to their organizational responsibilities in their interactions with patients. Following from Goffman's (*The presentation of self in everyday life*, Random House, 1959) frontstage/backstage dichotomy, this chapter addresses how interactional practices often involve attending to organizational responsibilities and how this 'backstage' work gets accomplished in 'frontstage' interactions. In outpatient settings, the 'backstage' practice of interacting with patients' electronic medical records overlaps with provider–patient interactions; in inpatient settings, the 'backstage' organizational work involves efforts at coordinating care with other providers, family members, and outside organizations, all of which reflects an NP's professional competency during 'frontstage' encounters.

Keywords Medical checklist • Electronic medical records • Coordinating care • Computer prompts

1 Introduction

Svennevig, in his discussion of leadership in workplace settings, points out that "some rights and obligations may be grounded in institutional structures, such as job descriptions and organizational routines, but they are also established and negotiated in actual communicative events" (2011, p. 19). In the case of medical visits, including those described in this book, some aspects of the interaction between provider and patient are based on 'institutional structures,' such as the need for nurse practitioners (NPs) to interact with a patient's electronic medical records (EMRs) during the visit or the need to coordinate care with other providers in order to deliver quality inpatient care. In this chapter, I discuss the ways in which competency is enacted through the fulfillment of particular organizational responsibilities and the utilization of organizational resources. Addressing organizational responsibilities has been given less scholarly attention in the medical discourse research in terms of how this may play a role in the provider–patient interaction, thereby limiting our understanding of how providers must balance multiple goals within an individual visit. Following Goffman's (1959) frontstage/backstage dichotomy, I argue that attending to organizational responsibilities gets enacted in the 'frontstage' but reflects 'backstage' practices. Therefore, viewing the fulfillment of organizational responsibilities as a part of what it means to be a competent provider sheds light on many of the linguistic choices NPs make. This is discussed in terms of the ways that NPs working in the outpatient Veterans Affairs (VA) clinic interact with patients' EMRs, a requirement of the organization, while also interacting with patients, and in how June, the NP working in an inpatient setting, makes a reference to her efforts at coordinating care with other providers as part of her interactions with patients. This analysis illustrates how NPs may bring their backstage work into the frontstage region of the medical visit as part of their enactment of professional competency.

2 Frontstage/Backstage in Professional Discourse

Researchers focusing on language use in professional settings have utilized Goffman's (1959) notion of the frontstage and the backstage, which has proven to be quite appropriate in descriptions of professional communication (Schnurr, 2013), workplace discourse (Koester, 2010), and medical discourse (Sarangi & Roberts, 1999). For Goffman, the frontstage, also referred to as the front region, is where performances in front of an audience occur; the backstage, or back region, is expected to not be seen by the audience. Using the metaphor of a stage performance, backstage is where rehearsals happen, where costumes and props are stored, where "flaws" (112) are hidden from view. The backstage work is hidden, contributing to "impression management" (113) and making it seem as though the frontstage performance is effortless. Goffman acknowledges that frontstage and backstage are often adjacent so that performers may get direction from someone backstage during a performance but that "the back region will be the place where the performer can reliably expect that no member of the audience will intrude" (113). Although this is also the case with medical visits in that patients are not present in laboratories nor do they typically have access to providers' notes that are shared electronically, medical providers may be required to share some of their backstage practices with patients or may choose to do so. In doing so, their backstage practices highlight and contribute to their performance of professional competency by revealing the work that gets accomplished on the part of the patient, beyond his/her individual medical encounter.

Schnurr (2013), Sarangi and Roberts (1999), and Koester (2010) all employ Goffman's frontstage/backstage metaphor in their description of professional communication. The most extensive discussion of the frontstage/backstage dichotomy is in Sarangi and Roberts' (1999) edited volume, *Talk, Work and Institutional Order*, where they argue that backstage interactions are just as integral to the study of workplace discourse as frontstage interactions and include a number of chapters that focus on backstage encounters between medical providers (c.f. chapters by Atkinson; Cook-Gumperz & Messerman; and Hall, Sarangi & Slembrouch (1999)). Sarangi and Roberts (1999) even suggest that what is typically considered frontstage (i.e. the provider–patient interaction) could be considered backstage, depending on the analytical focus. This 'blurring' (23) of frontstage and backstage is highlighted in Cook-Gumperz and Messerman's (1999) analysis of case meetings in which medical records are jointly constructed. In this study, the case meetings themselves are viewed as the frontstage and the provider–patient interactions are backgrounded, providing support for the provider–provider interactions. Despite this attention to the backstage work of medical discourse, in this study and others, the division of frontstage and backstage is kept distinct for the most part. In his argument for the need to study backstage encounters, Atkinson states that "the prominence of the primary medical encounter *masks* the variety of work and talk that are accomplished elsewhere– in the laboratories, in the specialist consulting services, and on such occasions as grand rounds, teaching rounds and the like" (1999, p. 76, emphasis added). While this seems to be true to a certain extent, there are also places not just where the concepts of frontstage and backstage are 'blurred,' but where they *bleed* into one another. By bleed, I am suggesting that the work that is done backstage becomes part of the provider–patient interaction, making it an integral component of the frontstage performance. Sarangi and Roberts acknowledge that "frontstage interactions are increasingly seen as contingent on backstage interactions" (1999, p. 24); however, studies have not highlighted the ways in which this is evident in the encounters in either the frontstage or backstage regions.

This chapter focuses on frontstage encounters between NPs and patients, addressing how backstage work is referenced and sometimes even accomplished in frontstage encounters, underscoring how attending to backstage, organizational responsibilities is part of the performance of professional competency. Although there are many ways in which providers may enact their professional competency through attending to frontstage and backstage concerns, in this chapter, I focus on two key components: attending to EMRs and coordinating care with other providers. Unlike the rest of the book, this chapter addresses organizational responsibilities in inpatient and outpatient visits separately, noting differing backstage forces influencing NPs' interactions with patients. First, in the VA outpatient clinic, NPs are required to engage with patients' EMRs during medical visits. Prompts in the EMR system direct much of the talk that occurs; therefore, considering how the EMR system plays a role in the encounter may shed light on some of the interactional choices that NPs make. Second, in the inpatient hospital setting, NPs often work in teams or units and must coordinate with other providers including the nurses working in the hospital and specialists who may have more limited interactions with the patients. Although most of this coordination happens backstage, it is important to acknowledge it during frontstage encounters as it reveals to patients the team approach that providers take and the work that they accomplish beyond the individual medical visit. Here, I focus not on the interactions that happen backstage, but how the backstage work gets enacted in the frontstage of medical encounters between NPs and patients.

The remainder of this section will address how attending to EMRs and coordinating care, both recognized as important components in the delivery of medical care, are a way in which the backstage bleeds into the frontstage.

2.1   EMRs and the Medical 'Checklist'

EMRs have become more ubiquitous in the United States, where their usage has doubled from 2008 to 2015 with over 80% of office-based physicians using them (Office of the National Coordinator for Health Information Technology, 2016). Because of this, EMRs play a greater role in how providers interact with patients during a medical visit. As an anecdote, I recently visited a provider, who rather than speak to me directly about his diagnosis and treatment plan, spoke the plan into the EMR system using speech-to-text software. He explained to me that this is how he copes with the requirements on his practice to keep detailed notes in this electronic format, and by reading them out in front of the patient, he can ensure that the patient gets the same information, at the same time. I include this example, not to criticize the provider but simply to highlight the very real ways that electronic records are changing the ways that healthcare providers practice medicine. Greatbatch (2006), in a study focused on prescribing practices by medical doctors, describes how these prescribing practices are influenced by the computer's presence in the room. By comparing the use of written prescription pads and prescriptions that are electronically entered on a computer, Greatbatch notes that the use of the computer, what he terms "text-based tasks," often interferes or overrides talk-based tasks (i.e. interacting with the patient). He includes interactional differences such as interrupting the talk to attend to computer-based prompts as well as giving patients information that is primed by the computer, essentially sharing with patients the more technical information as they enter it. He claims, in these cases, "the competencies involved in the accomplishment of text-based tasks are in many cases inseparable from those which underpin the doctor-patient interaction" (339), suggesting that the role of the provider is changing, which, in turn, changes the way that talk is accomplished in medical visits. In an in-depth study of the use of EMRs during medical visits, Soudi (2013) argues that the computer in the room should be considered a "third party," akin to an additional person present, as it "performs actions and contributes to the topics of development mainly through on-screen prompts" (35). Not only does the provider need to address his/her talk to the computer, but as Greatbatch notes, the computer plays a role in controlling the interaction, mainly through the on-screen prompts and a "set of reminders to ensure that the physician does not overlook any health complications or questions" (35). Although neither Soudi nor Greatbatch make the connection to backstage practices, it is reasonable to equate the use of the computer to something similar to other 'backstage' practices. It is comparable to Cook-Gumperz and Messerman's (1999) analysis of how written medical records are negotiated between providers in the backstage setting of weekly patient care meetings in that the computer is part of the organizational requirements and part of how patients' records are shared among providers, pharmacists, and other staff members. Because EMRs, which are a new way to create medical records, are institutionally incorporated in the patient–provider interaction, they are one of the ways in which the backstage work bleeds into frontstage spaces and influences the talk that occurs there.

As both Soudi and Greatbatch note, EMRs provide prompts for providers, guiding the questions they ask and the order in which they ask them. Seen in this light of 'structuring' the medical visit, the use of the computer and the interaction with the patient's EMRs is not so different from the practice that Boyd and Heritage (2006) describe for medical visits in which computers are not present. They note that the history-taking phase of the medical visit "usually involves moving through a set of routine, standardized questions" (2006, pp. 168–169), suggesting that providers are following a type of 'checklist,' which "may arise from record-keeping protocols, or from routine experience of the doctor, or from explicit guidelines taught during residency" (168). In the case of the VA outpatient visits, this 'checklist' is dictated by the organization and carried out through a series of computer prompts (personal communication). Following the 'checklist' and computer prompts is a way of conforming to organizational policies and expectations, an integral part of part of what it means to be a competent provider.

2.2 *Coordinating Care*

In addition to attending to a patient's EMR and the prescribed checklist, the NPs in this study enact their professional competency through coordinating care, an important part of successful healthcare delivery for providers working in any setting. Although there are many definitions of coordination of medical care, all reference the ways in which a patient's information is shared between different providers. O'Malley and Cunningham define it as the "degree to which information from various sources is recognized and incorporated into a patient's current care" (2009, p. 170). Some definitions also make reference to the inclusion of family members in the patient's care plan (Stille, Jerant, Bell, Meltzer, & Elmore, 2005), suggesting that coordination of care involves other entities who can provide support to patients. Stille and colleagues also make the distinction between collaboration and coordination. They argue:

> Collaboration is simply the act of working together, whereas coordination involves regulation of participants to produce higher-order functioning. It requires developing and guiding a therapeutic plan and integrating the inputs of multiple clinicians, patients, and families (and, at times, community agencies, employers, or schools) toward a common goal. (Stille et al., 2005, p. 700)

Stille and colleagues also note that coordinated care involves making explicit to patients exactly who is involved in their care—that is, informing patients about other team members and the roles they play.

Specific to inpatient diabetes care, Ross et al. (2014) discuss the role of diabetes specialist nurses (DSNs) in the United Kingdom in the coordination of care among other hospital staff. DSNs play a role quite similar to June's (the NP in this study working in an inpatient setting), in terms of providing patient education, coordination with dieticians, medical doctors, and other nursing staff members. In this study, the researchers identified key challenges to providing inpatient diabetes care to patients, including "allocating and managing a finite set of organizational resources including equipment; staff time and availability; physical space; and procedures and documents" (Ross et al., 2014, p. 96). They conclude that coordination of diabetes care is centrally performed by the diabetes specialist nursing team and involves coordination "vertically through the hierarchy of the organization, laterally between domains and specialties and longitudinally, to ensure that knowledge about the patient state is continually updated and monitored" (99). This is the case for June as well. As the data below illustrate, June continually coordinates care with other members of her team, including the dietician, a key component in diabetes education, and the endocrinologist, a specialist who often takes the lead in determining insulin dosages for patients. She also coordinates care with patients' family members to ensure that they are also knowledgeable and able to provide help to the patients upon discharge.

Although attending to EMRs and coordinating care are just two ways in which the NPs attend to their professional and organizational responsibilities, they highlight the work that providers engage in through backstage, organizationally defined job requirements, as well as the ways in which the backstage work bleeds into the frontstage setting of patient visits. The following section presents examples in which these backstage organizational practices get enacted during interactions with patients and considers how this work both influences the talk that occurs between provider and patient, as well as highlights their professional competency, illustrating to patients the multiple layers of care that their 'team' is able to provide.

3 Enacting Organizational Responsibilities

In this section, I focus first on the ways in which the institutionally dictated checklist plays a role in the structure and content of the medical visits in the VA outpatient clinic. I illustrate how both Karen, an NP working in primary care in the VA clinic, and the patient orient to the 'checklist' by focusing on the question and answer sequences. The second excerpt, also involving Karen, follows the same questioning format; however, in this one, she deviates from the checklist much more as new information is shared by the patient. Rather than simply checking boxes and confirming information, Karen's deviations, albeit brief, can be understood as adding to the patient's record as well as seeking clarification on new information. In both of these examples, it is clear that Karen is following the organizational requirements of attending to the patient's EMRs and addressing the computer prompts in the order that they are presented. From these excerpts, it is clear that the organizational requirements of updating the patients' EMRs—what might be seen as 'backstage' work—get done in frontstage interactions.

The second set of excerpts (3–6) address June's performance of professional competency in the inpatient setting by showing how June references her work of coordinating care with other providers in her interactions with patients. This is seen in her references to making arrangements for the dietician to come visit the patient (excerpt 3); referencing the work that other providers in her team do (excerpt 3–4); coordinating care with clinics outside the hospital (excerpt 5); and attempting to coordinate her visits with a patient's family members (excerpt 6). In each of these cases, June makes it explicit that (1) she is not the sole provider attending to the patient's care, but that there is a team, often working and communicating 'backstage,' to ensure quality care for patients and (2) she continues to work on behalf of the patient beyond her interactions with them. In doing so, she brings the backstage into the front region.

3.1 Attending to the Checklist

As described earlier, the history-taking/examination phase of primary care visits often follow what has been described as a checklist. As Boyd and Heritage (2006) illustrate, during this phase of the visit, both patients and providers orient to this checklist of questions. Providers do so by keeping their questions brief, designing them for optimal responses (i.e. showing a preference toward healthy rather than unhealthy habits) and with sensitivity toward the participant (i.e. acknowledging known information); in turn, patients orient to the checklist by keeping their responses brief and on topic. In the case of the outpatient VA visits, providers are given a 'checklist' of questions on their computer screen in which they must enter information so it can become part of the patient's record. Through the computer system, they also reorder prescriptions, schedule consultations with specialists, or order additional tests. The computer system dictates the 'checklist' of questions (Soudi, 2013); however, as Boyd and Heritage (2006) also note, the checklist is sometimes deviated from. In the case of the VA visits, NPs both follow the 'checklist' script that the computer system provides and allow deviations from the script when a patient shares information that may be pertinent to his/her health.

3.1.1 Good, and Uh, Any Heartburn?

The first excerpt is taken from a visit between Karen and Mr. Eggers. Mr. Eggers has been a patient of Karen's for many years, and unlike many of the patients she sees, Mr. Eggers does not have a private doctor outside the VA system. For this reason, Mr. Eggers comes in multiple times per year, although this visit is Mr. Eggers' annual check-up, where Karen asks about Mr. Eggers' ongoing medical issues and reviews any medications he is currently taking. The following excerpt occurs approximately two minutes into the visit and is fairly representative of the type of interaction that happens throughout this and many outpatient visits in which both provider and patient orient to the medical checklist.

Excerpt 1

1. Karen: how much metformin are you taking
2. Mr. Eggers: once a day half in the morning half in the evening
3. Karen: oh you're taking half and half?
4. Mr. Eggers: yeah
5. Karen: okay and how's that working
6. Mr. Eggers: can't complain
7. Karen: good (1.0) and uh (.) any <u>heart</u>burn or anything like that
8. Mr. Eggers: I still get the heartburn and stuff like that
9. Karen: are you still taking the ↑ premisol
10. Mr. Eggers: yeah but I mean (.) you're gonna get that for the most
11. part no
12. Karen: (1.0) um okay perfect what did you weigh today one
13. ninety-<u>four</u> so you <u>gained</u> five pounds
14. Mr. Eggers: yeah but I've lost I mean <u>last</u> week I weighed a hundred
15. and what ninety-<u>two</u> when I got my shot (.) my injection
16. Karen: oh yeah so how is your <u>knee</u> So they put it in your ↑ right
17. knee
18. Mr. Eggers: ahh yeah
19. Karen: okay
20. Mr. Eggers: it still needs to be replaced but I keep as long as the shots
21. work I-
22. Karen: and they just gave you one in November right
23. Mr. Eggers: yeah
24. Karen: November <u>tenth</u>
25. Mr. Eggers: November tenth and what was the last one April fifteenth
26. something like that (1.5) the shots do pretty good
27. Karen: <u>yes</u> I saw the one from April fourteenth right (.) okay (.)
28. good how is the numbness and tingling to your feet
29. Mr. Eggers: you know actually it's better

This excerpt begins with Karen asking Mr. Eggers about one of his current medications, metformin (line 1). Although Mr. Eggers responds with a seemingly dispreferred response on Karen's part, marked by her surprise ("oh") and repetition of his response ("you're taking half and half") in line 3, she does not inquire as to why he is taking this smaller dosage. She does follow up by asking if it is working for him (line 5) but then shifts to the next topic of heartburn, seeking information on a change in the state of his health since the previous visit. This pattern continues throughout the exchange. Attending closely to the computer-initiated checklist echoes what Mehan refers to as the IRE (Initiate, Respond, Evaluate) pattern of classroom discourse in which the teacher asks a question (or Inquires), the students Respond, and the teacher provides an Evaluation (cited in Cazden & Beck, 2008). Karen initiates a question, Mr. Eggers responds, and then Karen evaluates his response. Although her final responses do have an evaluative stance including "good" (lines 7 & 28), "perfect" (line 12), or "okay" (lines 5, 12, 17 & 27), these seem to be more of acknowledgment tokens than truly evaluative assessments of his responses (Atkinson, 1982). Other medical discourse researchers have also noted this three-part pattern (Atkinson, 1982; Mishler, 1984), arguing that it is a way to maintain control over the conversation and a reflection of the asymmetrical power inherent in medical visits. Although this may be true, there is more to this interactional practice than simply providers controlling talk. By viewing the checklist three-part sequence as a requirement of the organization, it becomes a more complicated picture and one that does not necessarily point to a provider's desire to control the talk but a way of balancing the organizational responsibilities with attending to the patient's needs.

It is true that Karen does not ask many follow-up questions or engage in any additional information that Mr. Eggers provides, even when the response he gives or the topic she initiates may seem less than ideal from a medical standpoint. This is the case with the discussion of heartburn in which he states that he does still get heartburn (line 8) as well as her mention of his five-pound weight gain (lines 12–13). Rather than expanding on these topics, she instead moves through the computer prompts addressing medication (lines 1 & 9), prior medical conditions (heartburn, line 7; numbness and tingling, line 28), timing of injections in his knee (22 & 24), and his weight (12–13).

I point out Karen's lack of topic expansion not to illustrate her lack of competence or her desire to control the talk. Based on her interactions with other patients, it is clear that when new or problematic answers arise, she addresses them, as will be shown in the following excerpt. It is likely, then, that because she knows Mr. Eggers well and because she does not find anything concerning in his answers, she is simply following the checklist, ensuring that there are no major changes in his health status. This excerpt shows how Karen strictly follows the checklist and is more focused on the institutional, backstage requirement of her role during her interaction with the patient. In what follows, I show how the backstage and frontstage get more blended as she deviates from the checklist as new information is introduced.

3.1.2 But Was He a Smoker?

The next excerpt illustrates how Karen continues to follow the checklist provided by the computer system but asks follow-up questions and allows topic deviation, particularly when new information arises. The patient, Mr. Franklin, has also been a patient of Karen for a number of years but sees her only once a year for his annual visit. As is mentioned in the excerpt, Mr. Franklin has a provider outside the VA system whom he sees more regularly. When this is the case, Karen is not only responsible for following the prompts based on his prior visit with her, but also adding any information that arises regarding changes in his health status since the last visit. Because of this, there are more topic deviations in this excerpt compared to the prior one.

Excerpt 2

1. Karen: you're not drinking anymore?
2. Mr. Franklin: oh no no I never dranked [does it say that on there
3. Karen: [okay good no it
4. [says none it says none
5. Mr. Franklin: [no I don't drink at all [I mean at all
6. Karen: [good good is your father
7. still alive
8. Mr. Franklin: yeah
9. Karen: how old is he now
10. Mr. Franklin: he's almost eighty seventy-seven but here's he
11. was I think I inherited some of this he was always
12. short (.) [winded
13. Karen: [of breath but he was a smoker?
14. Mr. Franklin: no [never smoked a Baptist minister never
15. Karen: [no oh really
16. Mr. Franklin: smoked a day in his life but, (.) forty years in the
17. mills
18. Karen: oh yeah the mills
19. Mr. Franklin: he worked at Kline's [(.) you know so
20. Karen: [okay so what are you doing
21. for your breathing medicines,
22. Mr. Franklin: I got the air (.) oh Doctor Burton gave me the air,

23.   I got the air at the house,
24. Karen: the what?
25. Mr. Franklin: the air
26. Karen: ↑ oxygen
27. Mr. Franklin: oxygen I'm sorry
28. Karen: you're wearing ↑ oxygen
29. Mr. Franklin: well yeah, he thought I don't really need it but he
30.   thought I did so I got everything they came by
31.   one day in a van and dropped off all kinds of- (.)
32. Karen: when are you wearing the oxygen?
33. Mr. Franklin: when I sleep sometimes I forget
34. Karen: okay
35. Mr. Franklin: and then it falls down on my nose
36. Karen: oh I know
37. Mr. Franklin: how are you supposed [to keep
38. Karen: [you have to just
39.   [tighten it around your ear yeah it's hard so and
40. Mr. Franklin: [I try but sometimes I wake up
41. Karen: what else are you- you got oxygen what else are
42.   you still taking the stomach pill from me
43. Mr. Franklin: yeah
44. Karen: have you had any ↑ heartburn
45. Mr. Franklin: ah no [no there ###
46. Karen: [okay are you still takin' the blood pressure
47.   medication,
48. Mr. Franklin: yep
49. Karen: a half tablet,
50. Mr. Franklin: yep

In the visit between Karen and Mr. Franklin, she follows the 'checklist' through her reliance on short, medical, and family-history-related questions. For example, in line 1, she asks him, displaying an optimization bias (Boyd & Heritage, 2006) for a negative answer, "you're not drinking anymore?"[1] The question is framed with negative polarity, indicating a preference for a negative answer, and suggests a change in condition from a previously discouraged action of drinking alcohol to one of abstinence, evident from the use of "anymore." This type of question formation is very much in line with the framing of questions by providers that Boyd and Heritage (2006) describe as part of the 'checklist' of history-taking. There is a brief departure from the 'checklist' when Mr.

Franklin questions the information in his medical chart: namely, whether the chart suggests that he was, formerly, a drinker. Here, both the patient and provider orient to the computer and EMR, making reference to what it 'says.' Reference is made later in the visit to Karen's need to update information 'into the computer,' acknowledging her responsibility to the organization and to the patient to keep his medical records up to date.

After clearing up this confusion in lines 3–4, the NP then returns to the checklist in lines 6–7 and 9, asking about the patient's father as a way of confirming family history. The first major departure from the checklist occurs in line 10 when Mr. Franklin then provides more information than what was asked of him, drawing a similarity between his father's health and his own by explaining that like himself, his father "was always short winded." Karen allows this deviation from the 'checklist' format, likely interpreting Mr. Franklin's contribution as relevant to the reasons for his lung problems. Prior to this exchange, Mr. Franklin admitted that he was a smoker. Her question, regarding whether Mr. Franklin's father was also a smoker, can be viewed as an attempt at drawing a correlation between Mr. Franklin's habits and his father's. Although she is not correct in her assumption (noted by the assumption bias in her statement question), and as is revealed in lines 16–19, this health condition is likely caused by his work in the local steel 'mills,' this departure has the potential for revealing possible genetic/family history of pulmonary disease compared to environmental factors such as smoking or unhealthy working conditions.

Following the first departure, Karen then returns to the 'checklist' by asking about his "breathing medications" (line 21), which prompts the second major departure. In line 22, Mr. Franklin describes his use of oxygen, referring to it as "the air" (lines 22–23), which is not a direct response, as the question was specifically about "medications"; however, this is relevant information and new information to Karen. The departure begins by first clearing up the confusion regarding the patient's use of the term "the air." Karen's use of repetition and rising intonation in lines 24 and 26 suggest that this is new or surprising information for her. She then engages in this topic by asking more questions regarding his use of oxygen and adherence to it. This is an important departure and one where the patient is prompted by a checklist question to introduce new, relevant information. Karen engages in this departure as the use of oxygen is both new to her (i.e. prescribed by another provider) and likely will be included as part of his chart, which will then presumably become one of the questions she asks at the next visit—essentially constructing part of the 'checklist' for future visits. Mr. Franklin, in lines 30 and 31, begins telling about his experience when the oxygen was dropped off at his house. Unlike the other departures, Karen does not encourage this one, but instead quickly turns the discussion back to what is medically relevant, which is 'when' he uses the oxygen (line 32).

Throughout this exchange, Karen addresses the 'checklist' questions dictated by the computer prompts but allows departures from the checklist when new information is introduced. Mr. Franklin taking oxygen, for example, would not necessarily be in his VA medical records since it was recently prescribed by another other provider outside the VA. Instead, Karen asks more information so that she can record this new information in his records. By following the 'checklist,' she is enacting her "organizational and work-role competencies" (Kak, Burkhalter, & Cooper, 2001) by updating Mr. Franklin's chart with information deemed to be important. In addition, she uses her professional knowledge and understanding that delving deeper into a topic through accessing the patient's "lifeworld" (Mishler, 1984) may reveal significant health information while disallowing topics such as the van delivery of oxygen.

As the previous two excerpts show, one of Karen's job requirements is to review and contribute to the patient's EMRs, both during and after the visit. During the visit, this takes the form of following the computer prompt checklist, inquiring about medications and previous health concerns. Depending on the patient and the patient's responses to certain questions, she may simply address the questions, acknowledge the patient's answers, and move on to the next item, as she does with Mr. Eggers in the previous excerpt. However, when new information arises in the course of the checklist questioning, she may deviate from the checklist to inquire about new information, as is the case in the visit with Mr. Franklin. Although Karen controls the talk through the use of the three-part sequence of question, answer, acknowledgment, she does so as a result of her organizational responsibilities. NPs working in the VA are required to follow the computer prompts and contribute to patients' EMRs—not engaging in the questions that the computer prompts require would mean that Karen is failing to attend to the work that is required by her organization. In addressing the computer prompts, Karen fulfills her organizational responsibilities in the frontstage setting of the medical visit.

3.2 Coordinating Care

In the next set of excerpts, I focus on June's fulfillment of organizational responsibilities through a second tactic of blending backstage and frontstage, namely, through her efforts at coordinating care with patients. June, a diabetes specialist working in an inpatient setting, similarly makes reference to patients' electronic records (excerpt 3); however, much of what she does in the front region involves acknowledging the work that other providers on her team do and the interactions she has with them in backstage interactions as well as working to coordinate care for patients after they have been discharged from the hospital.

3.2.1 We Have the Endocrinologist/Let's Bring a Dietician

The following excerpt comes from a visit between June and Ms. Martin. Ms. Martin was diagnosed with diabetes when she was a child and has struggled with managing her diabetes for most of her life. June and Ms. Martin have not met before this visit; because of this, June addresses a number of different issues and makes reference to two different members on her team—the endocrinologist (a specialist focused on the endocrine system and hormones including insulin) and the dietician. In the case of the former, June references the work that the endocrinologist is doing for the patient; for the latter, she offers to schedule an appointment for Ms. Martin with the dietician—both of which highlight the team that June works with and the collaborative work she does for patients. The excerpt includes three parts: (1) a discussion of the endocrinologist and her role (lines 1–12); (2) a discussion of Ms. Martin's struggle with carbohydrate counting and June's efforts at education (lines 63–82); and (3) June's offer to bring a dietician in to speak with Ms. Martin (lines 95–98).

Excerpt 3

1. June: what I do with di- with the hospitalists is diabetes
2. management so if we didn't already have an endocrinologist
3. on your case already I'd be picking doses for you
4. Ms. Martin: right
5. June: but we have the queen we have the expert we have the
6. endocrinologist already looking
7. Ms. Martin: right

8. June: her name is Dr. Jacobs and if you haven't met her you will
9. be meeting her and I suspect since we have the electronic
10. record she's actually choosing doses for you right now
11. Ms. Martin: right
12. June: and then is gonna make her way over here later in the day
... *(51 lines omitted)*
63. Ms. Martin: it's just sometimes I don't know how big the portion
64. should be of how much there should be
65. June: okay
66. Ms. Martin: and see a lot of the times there's a lot of times when we
67. have mashed potatoes and corn I know that's a lot of carbs
68. June: it's okay
69. Ms. Martin: you know and I try you know my portion that's my most
70. favorite
71. June: all right
... *(8 lines omitted)*
79. June: and if you want mashed potatoes and corn and birthday
80. cake have it because you're a carb counter there's no reason
81. that you can't cover your food because you're dosing
82. according to what you eat
... *(13 lines omitted)*
95. June: I think what I'm gonna do is if there's one thing I can be
96. of help is let's bring a dietician to talk about those carb
97. servings again that you can nail it down and get that
98. refresher course on what that food looks like

In the first part of the excerpt, June makes reference to the work that she usually does for patients through the use of the hypothetical statement, "if we didn't have the endocrinologist on your case already, I would be picking doses for you." In making this statement, June communicates one of her primary roles in the hospital, which is to select insulin doses for patients, highlighting her expertise and knowledge. In addition, she makes it clear that she has knowledge about Ms. Martin's 'case,' namely, that the endocrinologist is working on her insulin. Since this is the first mention of the endocrinologist in this visit, this information did not come from the patient; instead, June had this information prior to meeting with Ms. Martin, likely from reading her electronic records (referenced in lines 9–10), which include other providers' notes. In doing this, June references the backstage work that she does; in this instance, it is reviewing the patient's chart before meeting with her and knowing that Ms. Martin has yet to meet with the endocrinologist, Dr. Jacobs. Additionally, in line 10, by describing the work that Dr. Jacobs is doing for Ms. Martin "right now," June essentially acts as Dr. Jacobs' proxy, sharing information on her behalf in order to let the patient know that work is being done behind the scenes, outside of any given provider–patient interaction. In this way, June brings Dr. Jacobs' backstage work into her own frontstage interaction with Ms. Martin.

In the second part of the excerpt, Ms. Martin expresses her biggest concern in managing her diabetes, which is choosing the right foods and in the right portions (lines 63–70). June offers support to Ms. Martin in the form of comfort ("it's okay," line 68) and education (lines 79–82). This education extends beyond the excerpt presented here, but it is clear that June is fulfilling her organizational and professional responsibilities by educating patients, a topic that will be addressed more fully in the next chapter. June also offers, at the end of the excerpt (lines 95–98), to schedule a time for the dietician to meet with Ms. Martin to more fully address her dietary questions.

With Ms. Martin, June's role is diminished in some way by the inclusion of the endocrinologist working on the team. Despite this change in her role, June still fulfills her organizational responsibilities by sharing information with the patient regarding other members of the team. Much in the way that the DSNs in Ross et al.'s (2014) study coordinate care across different provider types, June plays a key role in coordinating care for the patients. Since the endocrinologist does not work onsite as June does, she explains the role that Dr. Jacobs is playing from her offsite office, highlighting the team aspect of Ms. Martin's care. This is reinforced in June's offer to bring in the dietician to talk to Ms. Martin, another important provider who can address Ms. Martin's specific concerns. By referencing the work that Dr. Jacobs does on Ms. Martin's behalf as well as efforts that June will make to coordinate care with the dietician on the team, June brings the backstage work of the hospital team into the frontstage. This foregrounding of backstage work is a way for June to enact her professional competency by showing the patient some of the work that happens outside of her interaction, giving the patient the impression that her care is being managed through a coordinated team effort.

3.2.2 That's What Kim Said

The second excerpt involving June takes place with a different patient, Mr. Clark. Mr. Clark has been hospitalized for three days at this point and June has met with him several times. This meeting is rather short, as June is simply checking in and discussing insulin adjustments with him. Although this is a fairly short visit, in it, she communicates to Mr. Clark that she is part of a team with many people working behind the scenes. This is evident in her reference to his conversation with the endocrinologist and information she received from one of the nurses, Kim.

Excerpt 4

1. June: and I suspected it wasn't doing a very good job for you
2. Mr. Clark: I agree with you
3. June: yeah and so I think we got all the confirmation we need and
4. I'd like to do what the endocrinologist spoke to you about
5. and take you off of seventy-five twenty-five and send you
6. home on two different kinds of insulin so you ate well last
7. night sir for supper
8. Mr. Clark: I always eat good
9. June: that's what Kim said good

Similar to the previous exchange between June and Ms. Martin, June references the endocrinologist on her team and the role that she plays in the patient's care. Here, unlike before, she actually references a conversation between Mr. Clark and the endocrinologist. Although it is possible that June was present for that visit, it is unlikely since the providers in this team all visit patients individually, based on their own schedule and availability. By referencing this conversation between Mr. Clark and Dr. Jacobs, June highlights the team's effort at coordinating Mr. Clark's care and the role that each of them play. In this case, it seems as though June is making the decision on changing Mr. Clark's insulin ('I'd like to do' line 4), which is in line with the recommendation by Dr. Jacobs.[2] Similarly, in line 9, June refers to another member of the team, Kim. In response to his claim that he "always eat(s) good" (line 8), June confirms this by stating 'that's what Kim said' (line 9). Again, it is not clear where June got this information per se, but it was outside of this visit. Whether it was from a face-to-face conversation that June had with Kim or information that she read in the patient's

EMRs, June's reference to this "conversation" with Kim reinforces to Mr. Clark that there is 'backstage' communication behind the scenes taking place regarding his health. Referencing such backstage communication that occurs behind the scenes, June's backstage work bleeds into her frontstage interactions, highlighting this aspect of her enactment of professional competency.

3.2.3 We Can Do That Ahead of Time

The previous two excepts illustrate how June coordinates care with other providers on her team and, more specifically, how she shares this information with patients. The following excerpt shows how June coordinates care outside of her team and outside of the hospital. In this excerpt, Mr. Harris expresses his concern about June changing his medication and how he will be able to get that medication after he is released from the hospital. June explains that she can work with the clinic where he is currently getting his medication to ensure that he is able to get this new type of insulin as well.

Excerpt 5

1. Mr. Harris: um so how how are we gonna work this out since I live in
2. Duncan
3. June: what do you mean precisely how are we gonna work this out
4. Mr. Harris: how how how (1.0) uh (.) insulin um well I (.) uh (.) see I
5. really don't have I have financial assistance through
6. Duncan hospital but I don't know- don't have insurance
7. June: where are you getting the seventy thirty from sir
8. Mr. Harris: the free free samples from um (.) the nurses out there (.) at
9. the hospital (1.0) Dr. Roberts' nurses
10. June: and when you say at the hospital is that a clinic [in a hospital
11. Mr. Harris: [yeah well
12. it's a hospital clinic combined and I can get some
13. from him but the diabetes lady down there? Sally
14. Bowden (.) gave me uh (.) one free sample to get start
15. June: okay (*walks to board and starts writing*) what we're going
16. to do is (.) we're gonna get you on the right stuff to start with
17. Mr. Harris: mhm
18. June: and then you'll go home on the right stuff (.) the best
19. stuff and then we can do two different things (1.5) we can
20. figure out if (.) where you're getting the seventy thirty?

21.		<u>also</u> has those two drugs and we can do that ahead of time
22.		(.) with a phone call before you <u>leave</u>

The excerpt begins with Mr. Harris asking about how he will get the insulin that June wants to prescribe to him once he leaves the hospital. He is concerned because he does not have insurance, and although he has been able to get free medication from his local clinic (located approximately two hours away), he is unsure whether that will be the case with the new medication. June provides a solution to this, which is to contact the clinic and determine if they also carry the new medication (lines 19–22).[3] She uses the first-person plural pronoun, "we," (line 21) making it unclear whether June herself will contact that clinic or whether someone on her team will. Nevertheless, it is her position within this team and as the diabetes specialist to alleviate his concern and ensure that he can continue to get the best care or "the best stuff" (lines 18–19) after he goes home. Unlike in the previous excerpts, here, June references backstage work that will be done (i.e. making "a phone call") rather than backstage work that has been completed prior to the interaction.

3.2.4 The Nurse Can Always Page Me

This final example of June's efforts to coordinate care for patients occurs during a visit with Ms. Anderson, a patient who has been in the hospital for two days and, like many of the patients June sees, is concerned about what happens when she goes home. She previously mentioned that her husband and son were there visiting her but are not able to make it very often because of transportation issues. June then explains that she will make herself available to meet with Ms. Anderson's family the next time they are able to come. In this excerpt, it is clear that June is focused on bringing the family into the discussion of care, coordinating with them what support they can provide after Ms. Anderson leaves the hospital.

Excerpt 6

1.	June:	and if at any time you think that hubby or son can be
2.		here and they wanna hear it from me
3.	Ms. Anderson:	mhm
4.	June:	or we can have a three-way discussion the nurse can

```
 5.              always page me
 6. Ms. Anderson: okay
 7. June:         okay and then um sometimes Ms. Anderson I understand
 8.              transportation I'm also available to make a phone call
 9.              and answer any questions over the phone
10. Ms. Anderson: okay
11. June:         I find that the best success and really that's all I want
12.              for you is to be successful is if you have backup singers
```

In this excerpt, June references Ms. Anderson's family members (line 1) and the possibility of sharing information with them. She uses the vague phrase "hear it from me" (line 2), which references an earlier conversation regarding how to properly interpret blood sugar readings and select the correct dose based on that reading. June is worried about Ms. Anderson's ability to do this on her own as she has explained that she cannot see very well and that her husband provides a lot of support for her, both in administering her insulin shots and cooking for her, another important component of diabetes management. She offers her expertise either in person by having the nurse page her (lines 4–5) or by calling them (lines 8–9), underscoring her efforts at coordinating care for patients beyond working with other providers on her team to working with families as well, as Stille et al. (2005) suggest.

4 Conclusion

Fulfilling organizational responsibilities takes many different forms in healthcare delivery. As researchers such as Atkinson (1999) and Cook-Gumperz and Messerman (1999) show, much of this work takes place backstage in intraprofessional interactions from which the patient is often excluded. Although it is important to acknowledge the backstage interactions, particularly in our collective understanding of medical discourse and professional communication in healthcare settings, it is important to also note how this backstage works bleed into the frontstage interactions between provider and patient. Rather than seeing these as completely separate parts of what it means to perform professional competency, this chapter highlights how the backstage aspect of professional competency is enacted in the 'front region.' It was shown that such backstage work is brought into frontstage interactions through

(1) attending to patients' EMRs and working through the organizationally defined 'checklist' and (2) by highlighting teamwork that occurs behind the scenes.

In the case of Karen and other NPs working in the outpatient VA clinic, the EMRs act as a third party in the medical visits (Soudi, 2013), dictating topics and even the order that topics are introduced. Although NPs are required to follow the computer prompts, they also are willing to deviate from those prompts when necessary. In doing so, they are also contributing to the patient's medical records by adding new information as they go. Karen, the NP working in the VA outpatient clinic, also makes a brief reference to her backstage work of inputting information into the patient's record after the visit, communicating with the patient the backstage work that she does even after the visit is over.

June, while also interacting with patients EMRs throughout her day, does so behind the scenes, or backstage. However, she uses this information to highlight her knowledge of the patients' care and to share with patients the efforts that are being made behind the scenes on their behalf, bringing the backstage into the frontstage. Similar to the description of diabetes specialist nurses in the United Kingdom that Ross et al. (2014) describe, June appears to be one of the primary contact persons for the patient. She is present even when the endocrinologist is working offsite and is able to share information with the patients on the work that is being done on their behalf. She also references other members on her team and coordinates care with other clinics and with family members.

Although the organizational responsibilities in these two healthcare settings are different, the excerpts in this chapter illustrate how these responsibilities, some of which are primarily performed backstage, bleed into frontstage interactions. In Goffman's discussion of frontstage and backstage, he argues that the backstage area in many settings is intended to be hidden from the audience. He gives the example of a hotel or a funeral home, in which it might be upsetting for the 'audience' to see what happens behind the scenes. In the case of the medical visits described here, it is more likely the case that there is comfort in knowing at least some of the work that happens in the backstage region. By referencing this backstage work as a performative act in the frontstage region, NPs are able to highlight their professional competency in terms of providing care for patients beyond the individual visit.

NOTES

1. Karen's formulation seems to suggest that Mr. Franklin was formerly a drinker but had stopped at some point in the past. As the transcript indicates, the notes in the EMR simply state 'none.' One of the critiques of EMRs, by providers, is that they often do not offer space for elaboration or notes (personal communication). This may be case here as Karen either confuses Mr. Franklin with another patient or makes an assumption that he previously drank, and without the opportunity to include these types of notes in his EMR, she only has the word 'none' to rely on. Further, because she only sees him once a year, it is likely that she would not remember details of prior conversations with him.
2. The use of 'we' in line 3 could also reference the team ('we got all the confirmation we need'). As discussed in Defibaugh (2014), the use of second-person plural pronouns often have the effect of bringing the patient into the decision-making process. It is unclear, here, whether the 'we' refers to June and Mr. Clark, June and Dr. Jacobs, or all three.
3. In line 19, June suggests that there are 'two different things' she can do to address Mr. Harris' prescription needs; however, the conversation moves away from this topic and she never returns to the second option; therefore, it is unclear what her alternate solution is.

REFERENCES

Atkinson, J. M. (1982). Understanding formality: The categorization and production of 'formal interaction. *British Journal of Sociology, 33*(1), 86–117.

Atkinson, P. (1999). Medical discourse, evidentiality, and the construction of professional responsibility. In S. Sarangi & C. Roberts (Eds.), *Talk, work, and institutional order* (pp. 75–108). Berlin: Mouton de Gruyter.

Boyd, E., & Heritage, J. (2006). Taking the history: Questioning during comprehensive history-taking. In J. Heritage & D. W. Maynard (Eds.), *Communication in medicine* (pp. 151–184). Cambridge: Cambridge University Press.

Cazden, C., & Beck, S. (2008). Classroom discourse. In A. C. Graesser, M. A. Gernsbacher, & S. R. Goldman (Eds.), *Handbook of discourse processes* (pp. 165–198). Mahwah, NJ: Lawrence Erlbaum Publishers.

Cook-Gumperz, J., & Messerman, L. (1999). Local identities and institutional practices: Constructing the record of professional collaboration. In S. Sarangi & C. Roberts (Eds.), *Talk, work, and institutional order* (pp. 145–183). Berlin: Mouton de Gruyter.

Defibaugh, S. (2014). Solidarity and alignment in nurse practitioner/patient interactions. *Discourse & Communication, 8*(3), 260–277.

Goffman, E. (1959). *The presentation of self in everyday life*. New York: Random House.
Greatbatch, D. (2006). Prescriptions and prescribing: Coordinating talk- and text-based activities. In J. Heritage & D. W. Maynard (Eds.), *Communication in medicine* (pp. 313–339). Cambridge: Cambridge University Press.
Hall, C., Sarangi, S., & Slembrouck, S. (1999). The legitimation of the client and the profession: Identities and roles in social work discourse. In S. Sarangi & C. Roberts (Eds.), *Talk, work, and institutional order* (pp. 293–322). Berlin: Mouton de Gruyter.
Kak, N., Burkhalter, B., & Cooper, M. (2001). Measuring the competence of healthcare providers. *Operations Research Issue Paper, 2*(1). Bethesda, MD: Published for the U.S. Agency for International Development (USAID) by the Quality Assurance (QA) Project.
Koester, A. (2010). *Workplace discourse*. London: Continuum.
Mishler, E. (1984). *The discourse of medicine: Dialectics of medical interviews*. Norwood, NJ: Ablex.
O'Malley, A. S., & Cunningham, P. J. (2009). Patient experiences with coordination of care: The benefit of continuity and primary care physician as referral source. *Journal of General Internal Medicine, 24*(2), 170–177.
Office of the National Coordinator for Health Information Technology. (2016). Office-based Physician Electronic Health Record Adoption. *Health IT Quick-Stat No 50*. dashboard.healthit.gov/quickstats/pages/physician-ehr-adoption-trends.php
Ross, A. J., Anderson, J. E., Kodate, N., Thompson, K., Cox, A., & Malik, R. (2014). Inpatient diabetes care: Complexity, resilience and quality of care. *Cognition, Technology & Work, 16*(1), 91–102.
Sarangi, S., & Roberts, C. (1999). The dynamics of interactional and institutional orders in work-related settings. In S. Sarangi & C. Roberts (Eds.), *Talk, work, and institutional order* (pp. 1–57). Berlin: Mouton de Gruyter.
Schnurr, S. (2013). *Exploring professional communication: Language in action*. Abingdon, Oxon: Routledge.
Soudi, A. (2013). *Competing lines of action: A sociolinguistic approach to the human-computer interface in doctors' consultations*. Unpublished doctoral dissertation, University of Pittsburgh, Pittsburgh, PA.
Stille, C. J., Jerant, A., Bell, D., Meltzer, D., & Elmore, J. G. (2005). Coordinating care across diseases, settings, and clinicians: A key role for the generalist in practice. *Annals of Internal Medicine, 42*, 700–708.
Svennevig, J. (2011). Leadership style in managers' feedback in meetings. In J. Angouri & M. Marra (Eds.), *Constructing identities at work* (pp. 17–39). London: Palgrave Macmillan.

CHAPTER 3

Need to Know: Patient Education and Epistemic Responsibility

Abstract Patient education is one of the foundations for healthcare delivery. The ways in which information is shared with patients can determine how much information is retained (Kessels, *Journal of the Royal Society of Medicine, 96*(5), 219–222, 2003). When information is too technical, patients may not be able to recall that information later; however, when patient education is done effectively, it can have positive impacts on patients' health (Mazzuca et al., *Diabetes Care, 6*, 347–350, 1983; Orth et al., *Health Psychology, 6*, 29–42, 1987). This chapter considers how information is shared with patients by drawing on Stivers, Mondada, and Steensig's (Knowledge, morality and affiliation in social interaction. In *The morality of knowledge in conversation* (pp. 3–26), Cambridge University Press, 2011) dimensions of knowledge, suggesting that nurse practitioners prioritize patients' primacy or 'right to know' over assessing 'access' and address this primacy by making information comprehensible, primarily through the use of low-register terminology and drawing patients in to the process of information exchange.

Keywords Information sharing • Technical/nontechnical terminology • Epistemic access • Epistemic primacy • Medical expertise

1 Introduction

Patient education and knowledge sharing is a key aspect of medical care and one that is accomplished almost exclusively through linguistic means. In this chapter, I examine the ways in which nurse practitioners (NPs) decide what information to share with patients, when to share it, and in what form. Information sharing in this chapter is framed in terms of Stivers, Mondada, and Steensig's (2011) dimensions of knowledge. I argue that, unlike everyday conversations, medical interactions require that providers assess prior access to medical information in distinctly different ways, either by simply sharing it with them, regardless of whether this is new or repeated information, or by drawing on the context of the visit to determine the level of prior knowledge that patients display. More importantly, the NPs in this study seem to prioritize patients' primacy or 'rights to know' certain information over taking the time to assess prior knowledge. In doing so, NPs enact their professional competency through attending to their epistemic and professional responsibility by ensuring that the information they share is comprehensible and applicable to the patients. This is primarily accomplished through the use of simple formulations and low-register terminology. However, when patients themselves show a high level of knowledge and a willingness to learn more, NPs will shift strategies and employ more technical language, thereby adapting to the individual patient's needs.

2 Knowledge and Information Sharing in Medical Visits

The role of knowledge and information sharing in medical visits has been well documented with studies focusing both on the role that patient-sharing can play in the visit as well as the importance of knowledge sharing on the part of the provider. Roter and Hall (1992), in their discussion of the "communication transforming principles," note that communication should both "reflect the special expertise and insight that the patient has into his or her physical state and well-being" as well as "maximize the usefulness of the physician's expertise" (5). Research has attempted to highlight the value of both of these perspectives in terms of knowledge sharing and its relationship with quality health care.

A number of studies have pointed out that one of the ways in which patient-centered care can be enacted is through allowing patients to share their experiences. Frankel and Stein (1999), for example, include "elicit the patient's perspective" as one of the four components of their "Four Habits Model" (82). Others have highlighted the importance of tapping into the patient's experiences in the medical visit; Mishler (1984) refers to this as accessing the patient's "lifeworld"; Haidet and Paterniti (2003) suggest that providers engage in "narrative-based medicine," which involves the use of different linguistic techniques to elicit the patient's experience with a particular illness or set of symptoms. Although this aspect of the medical visit is important, the focus of this chapter is on knowledge sharing on the part of the provider, which is also an essential component of the patient-centered approach.

Focus on providers' knowledge has also been well documented in the research, noting that the ways and the extent in which providers share technical information is essential to effective healthcare delivery (Frankel & Stein, 1999) and often a delicate balancing act. As Waitzkin (1985) explains, providers "have the subtle responsibility of deciding how much information is in the patients' best interests" (81). Waitzkin (1985) and others (Charles, Gafni, & Whelan, 1997; Mooney & Ryan, 1993; Roter & Hall, 1992) have shown that patients typically want a greater amount of information, particularly about their diagnosis and treatment, than providers often offer. Mooney and Ryan (1993) point out that patients are looking for some kind of reassurance about their illness in order to reduce anxiety, which can be accomplished through information sharing. Patients' preference for a greater amount of information can also be seen in the ways that information sharing has been positively correlated with health outcomes and satisfaction (Beck, Daughtridge, & Sloane, 2002; Mazzuca, Weinberger, Kurpius, Froehle, & Heister, 1983; Orth, Stiles, Scherwitz, Hennrikus, & Vallbona, 1987). Mazzuca et al. (1983) noted greater comprehension rates of the need for individual agency and self-care among diabetes patients whose recent test results were explained to them. In a study of patients with a history of high blood pressure, Orth et al. (1987) found a positive correlation between lower blood pressure readings by patients during a home visit two weeks after the medical visit and the amount of explanation about high blood pressure by providers during the visit. These studies illustrate the importance of information sharing on the part of the provider in terms of positive health outcomes for patients.

As Roter and Hall argue, despite these positive outcomes, providers are not always effective at passing on their expert knowledge to patients, noting that providers often use technical terms that patients likely do not know and even use terminology during visits that they previously reported patients likely would not be familiar with (1992). It is clear from this study and those discussed earlier that one should not take for granted the importance of providing information to patients in ways that are clear and informative to them based on their particular illness, and as I will show, their current place of understanding and dealing with their illness. In this chapter, I focus on the ways in which information is shared with patients regarding treatment (excerpts 1 and 3) as well as more general information about the patient's condition (excerpts 2 and 4), primarily through the use of low-register, nontechnical terms that are accessible to patients but also by prioritizing certain information over others, based on the NPs' expert knowledge and experience.

2.1 Features of Information Sharing

As the previous section outlined, numerous researchers have noted the importance of information sharing. The basis of these studies is primarily from post-visit interviews and surveys, or in the case of Orth and colleagues, empirical data collection of blood pressure readings. Although these studies highlight the value of knowledge sharing, they do not necessarily address what this looks like in the medical visit. Waitzkin (1985) compares provider post-visit impressions of amount of time explaining and sharing information with patients with recordings of the medical visits. In this comparison, he notes that the physicians in his study greatly overestimate the amount of time they spend sharing information with patients, suggesting that providers are actually doing much less than what they believe they are doing. Although this study does not quite get to the linguistic characteristics of the explanations, it does shed light on the difference in provider perceptions and the quantifiable time spent on this aspect of the visit.

Heritage (2005) seeks to identify exactly what providers are doing when they share diagnostic information with patients. He draws on three studies spanning 20 years of provider–patient research, which focus on the diagnosis/treatment phase of the primary care visit. In each of these studies, the patient is seeking a diagnosis for an acute illness. The study of greatest relevance to this chapter is based on work by Peräkylä (1998). Heritage (2005) describes the three patterns of sharing diagnostic information that Peräkylä found: plain assertion, evidential, and evidence formulating. Plain assertion involves simply a statement of the diagnosis, while evidential and evidence formulating include an explanation of how the provider reached his/her diagnostic conclusion. Heritage's discussion (as well as Peräkylä's original study) of these three diagnosis styles sheds light on some of the ways providers use different linguistic means to share information with patients. Heritage notes that these styles highlight the provider's authority as a medical professional in making diagnostic claims as well as, in the case of evidential and evidence formulating, a sense of accountability or a need to justify their conclusions with patients. Heritage (2005) and Peräkylä's (1998) concept of authority and accountability in knowledge sharing is particularly relevant in the domain that they study—which is offering diagnoses. However, accountability may be less relevant in other realms of knowledge sharing in medical visits such as in education associated with disease management, in which the provider may feel less of a need to justify his/her professional expertise. One example of this, discussed below, is an explanation of how to lower cholesterol levels. Laura, the NP, does not need to justify how she came upon this information; instead, her role is to share commonly known information with the patients. This difference in information-sharing goals in such non-diagnostic aspects of medical visits can better be explained through the incorporation of Stivers, Mondada, and Steensig's (2011) "dimensions of knowledge" framework, which considers the negotiation of epistemic access, primacy, and responsibility between interlocutors.

2.2 Dimensions of Knowledge

Stivers, Mondada, and Steensig (2011) provide a framework for examining knowledge in everyday conversation. They claim that, "In conversation, interactants show themselves to be accountable for what they know, their level of certainty, their relative authority, and the degree to which they exercise their rights and fulfill their responsibilities" (9). Their focus is on the linguistic and interactional means in which knowledge is shaped through interaction. In putting forth their account of knowledge sharing in conversation, they outline three "dimensions of knowledge": epistemic access, epistemic primacy, and epistemic responsibility.

Epistemic access is conceived of in binary terms: one either has access to particular information or does not. They examine ways in which this access is negotiated, that is, how participants determine if a conversational partner has access to particular information, how one elicits access that information, and how one might claim his/her own access. Determining whether someone else has access to knowledge is a complex endeavor, as the authors point out. It is expected that conversational participants will not share information that is already known to others, making prefaces particularly important. They give the examples of prefacing information sharing with questions such as 'did I mention' or 'have I told you,' which allows speakers to determine if their interactional participants already have access to certain knowledge. In terms of claims, rather than inquiries of access, they argue that epistemic access can be claimed outright or downgraded through the use of hedging or mitigation devices (see Chap. 4 for more on this). It can be sought from another through direct questioning or request for information (i.e. request for access).

Unlike access, epistemic primacy is, by nature, scalable and unequal in terms of interactants' position with respect to one another. Primacy is concerned with who has the right to know as well as who has the right to inform. Stivers, Steensig, and Mondada (2011) give the example of a close friend finding out important news from a more distant friend or colleague as a violation of primacy in terms of who has a greater 'right to know.' They also argue that assertions should be made by those who have greater epistemic authority, which is "sometimes derivable from social categories" (16), as in the case of medical professionals compared to patients, and sometimes from interactional roles (i.e. the storyteller or direct experiencer of events). In the case of the latter, the interactional first turn, or initiator of the topic, often is a way for individuals to make a claim of epistemic primacy. When the position is a bit more contestable, speakers may use hedges or mitigation to soften their claim of primacy. It is important to note here that epistemic primacy includes both the concept of who has authority over particular information as well as who has a right to know that information. For the purposes of this chapter, I will use the term 'epistemic authority' for the former concept and 'epistemic primacy' for the latter. In the case of the excerpts discussed in this chapter, the NP has certain 'epistemic authority,' meaning greater access to medical knowledge; patients have a certain level of 'epistemic primacy' or right to know about their medical condition.

Epistemic responsibility is described by the authors as when interactants "attend not only to who knows what, but also to who has a *right* to know what, who knows *more* about what and who is *responsible* for knowing what" (18, emphasis in original). In that respect, epistemic responsibility can be understood as the management of access and primacy. Conversational participants are understood as being responsible for knowing what is 'common ground' or shared knowledge, and responsible for knowing who has access, and whether access is shared among participants. They are also responsible for attending to the primacy asymmetry in terms of both sharing what one knows that others may have a right to know and avoiding sharing knowledge when one is in a lower position of authority.

2.2.1 Dimensions of Knowledge, Authority, and Accountability in Medical Visits

These concepts, or dimensions of knowledge, as Stivers, Mondada and Steensig describe them, are key elements in understanding how knowledge is constructed in interaction. Although these authors are primarily concerned with (1) everyday interactions and (2) the interactional mechanisms in which knowledge is displayed, shared or contested in interactions, these concepts are well suited to an analysis of knowledge sharing in medical visits because they can help explain the choices that providers make in their choices of both *what* information to share and *when*, and *how* information is shared. In this chapter, I focus less on the interactional, turn-by-turn mechanisms of knowledge sharing and more on the ways in which NPs may prioritize one of these dimensions over others. It is also important to note that Stivers and colleagues are primarily concerned with everyday interactions in which there is not an institutional asymmetry that overlays the ways that knowledge is shared. Because of the contextual differences in their study and the present one, a few caveats are in order.

As Heritage and Clayman (2010) describe, institutional talk, such as provider–patient interactions, has distinct elements, including (1) "specific goal orientations *which are tied their* (participants) *institutional-relevant identities*" (34, emphasis in original); (2) particular constraints on the talk which are understood and "allowable," based on the institution and the goals associated with it; and (3) understood and agreed-upon procedures and shared ways of framing the interaction within the institutional context. All these features of institutional talk are important here as they contribute to an understanding of knowledge sharing in terms of access, primacy, and responsibility. Because medical visits are asymmetrical by nature, the way that knowledge is positioned within these visits is also asymmetrical in a way that it may not be in everyday talk. That is, the setting itself and the institutional roles determine who has access, primacy, and responsibility.

In a medical visit, the provider often has access to knowledge that patients do not necessarily have.[1] Medical providers are endowed with what Heritage (2005) refers to as "cultural authority" (84) in which providers are able to diagnose illnesses "based on special knowledge possessed and controlled by the profession of medicine" (85). Medical providers can be viewed as being part of an "epistemic community" (Holzner, 1968) in which they have greater privilege to knowledge within the medical domain or greater "epistemic authority." In the case of the excerpts discussed in this chapter, this greater epistemic authority is not limited only to the ability to diagnose and treat a particular condition, but to greater knowledge of what information might be more important for patients at particular moments (excerpt 1), how an illness works (excerpt 2), and what diagnostic and evaluative measures mean (excerpts 3–4).

Epistemic responsibility in this setting should also be understood within the framework of the institutional setting of the medical visit. Because of the high stakes of nature associated with medical knowledge (i.e. having relevant knowledge can be the difference between behavioral/health improvement and decline), and the inherent asymmetry of medical interactions, two basic premises require reanalysis of Stivers and colleagues' definition of "epistemic responsibility." The first is that it may be more important for a provider to share relevant knowledge rather than trying to assess whether the patient already has this information. One reason for this is the time limitations, which may encourage providers to favor assertions over an information-check style of questioning, which would naturally take more time. Additionally, unlike in everyday conversations, an information check to determine patients' epistemic access could be face threatening to them if they do not, in fact, have that information. Because the provider is in a higher position of authority and in a position to evaluate or judge patients' knowledge, patients may feel that they have failed in some way by either not having that information or not being able to access it in the moment. Therefore, telling, rather than asking, may be preferred in this setting. It is also important to note that the provider has a responsibility to share information in a way that patients can understand (Kessels, 2003; Roter & Hall, 1992). Studies have found, for example, that quasi-technical terms like 'hypertension' or 'obese' are defined differently by medical providers and lay persons (Hadlow & Pitts, 1991), pointing out the need for clarity in communication of medical terms and sharing of medical knowledge. As Roter and Hall explain, "physicians have the duty to share their medical expertise with patients in such a way that this information is clear, relevant, and useful to patients" (1992, p. 11). Therefore, 'epistemic responsibility,' in the case of medical visits, should be understood as the provider's obligation to share information with patients that they believe is integral to their health, regardless of whether they believe the patient may already know this information. Additionally, information should be shared in a way that patients can easily comprehend, thereby allowing patients better access to knowledge.

3 Prioritizing Patient's Primacy over Assessing Prior Access

The remainder of this chapter will focus on four data extracts in which the NPs manage their epistemic responsibility by providing patients with relevant knowledge needed to manage their current medical conditions. In doing so, they prioritize a patient's primacy, that is their "rights to know" (Stivers et al., 2011, p. 13) over assessing their access. The way that epistemic responsibility is enacted varies, depending on the context, the patient, and the topic. In the first two extracts, June relies on her prior experience with diabetes patients to foreground certain information that she deems most critical while backgrounding other information which may confuse the patient later. The second extract comes from the same visit; in this extract, June uses low-register, nontechnical terminology and invites the patient into the knowledge sharing process through the use of rhetorical questions. The third extract comes from an outpatient visit and also illustrates how the use of technical information is made accessible to the patient through the use of low-register terms. In this extract, the NP, Laura, 'translates' the patient's health data into specific food choices, bringing his daily habits into part of the information exchange, thereby making the information seem more personalized. Finally, in the fourth extract, I return to the work that June does in educating patients about diabetes and show that she adjusts her level of specificity and technical terminology based on the patients' current display of knowledge. Together, these examples illustrate a range of ways that NPs manage their epistemic responsibility in the medical visit. In the case of June interacting with Ms. Piper and Mr. Tucker, these examples also reveal how she evaluates patients' access and primacy and adjusts accordingly, attending to individual patient needs and current levels of knowledge.

3.1 It's in Your Best Interest to Get Out of the Big Numbers

The first excerpt is taken from a visit between June and Ms. Piper. Ms. Piper has been preliminarily diagnosed with diabetes, and in this first meeting between the two, June wants to assess what kind of aid Ms. Piper needs in dealing with her new diagnosis. The extract starts with June using a tactic she often employs with patients to elicit their primary concerns (lines 2–4). Ms. Piper hints that her concern is about having blood sugar levels that are too low, causing her to go into a diabetic coma. Although June listens to this concern, she redirects the discussion to what she views as the biggest concern for newly diagnosed individuals: having levels that are too high. In redirecting the conversation, June is positioning certain knowledge as being more important; she is also drawing on her own epistemic authority to address Ms. Piper's primacy, or right to know critical information for newly diagnosed diabetics.

Excerpt 1

1. June: so before I get started on those small (.) assignments or
2. what those assignments need to be: (1.0) what is your
3. most pressing concern angst fears worries freak out ↑
4. moments (0.5) as you think about being told in the
5. hospital that the blood sugars are too high and that they
6. are diagnosable for diabetes (3.0)
7. Ms. Piper: I guess (.) how to treat it I guess is my biggest concern um
8. (.) both my parents are diabetics (0.5) my mom actually
9. went into a diabetic coma (.) so (.) [it's a little
10. June: [from low from low
11. blood sugar
12. Ms. Piper: scary yeah
13. June: alright
14. Ms. Piper: I mean the EMTs said her blood sugar was twelve
15. June: okay very scary
16. Ms. Piper: yeah (1.0)
17. June: and you (.) have a ↑ child
...(*115 lines omitted*)
132. June: in fact because you've been living with a blood sugar of
133. three hundred even a normal blood sugar (.) might feel
134. crappy (.) and you check a blood sugar see if its ↑ low
135. and you'll be a lo:ng way from going into a coma
136. because we're gonna readjust your body from thinking
137. that three hundred is a good number (1.0) to down in

138.		those low (.) one hundreds being a good <u>number</u> and that
139.		doesn't happen immediately but you can see if you started
140.		feeling shaky sweaty symptoms of low blood sugars and
141.		you check and you're (.) one <u>eighty</u> (.) or one <u>fifty</u> (1.0)
142.		you're a lo::ng way from going into a <u>coma</u> (1.0) and
143.		that's that part of time where we have to get your body
144.		rea<u>djust</u>ed to what good numbers <u>are,</u>
145.	Ms. Piper:	so in essence the goal is to drop the numbers <u>slowly</u> I
146.		don't wanna just shwoot
147.	June:	(2.0) not exactly (1.0) no because it is in <u>best</u> interest to
148.		get the good numbers as soon as <u>poss</u>ible because
149.		you're in the hospital with <u>chest</u> pains #### so (.)
150.		be<u>cause</u> you're in an <u>acute</u> setting and be<u>cause</u> we have
151.		an <u>acute</u> need for good blood sugars, we're gonna use
152.		the <u>best</u> products and we're gonna get it down (.)
153.		we're gonna get it <u>down</u> as quickly as we can get
154.		it <u>down</u>=
155.	Ms. Piper:	=but i'm gonna feel yucky [in the meantime=
156.	June:	[you might =you
157.		might (1.0) just sayin' <u>hon</u>est [honest very honest
158.	Ms. Piper:	[mhm
159.	June:	with my patients (.) it's in your best interest to get
160.		out of the <u>big</u> numbers and you <u>might not</u> (.) feel
161.		great when you do it (1.0) you might feel symptoms
162.		of a low blood sugar, before you're really <u>low</u>
163.	Ms. Piper:	and symptoms of low blood sugar a:re:?
164.	June:	we'll get to that later let me tell you about your
165.		medicine now

The first part of the excerpt highlights Ms. Piper's concern, which is about having blood sugar levels that are too low that would cause her to go into a diabetic coma. She first frames here concern as "how to treat" diabetes (line 7). She then highlights her prior knowledge by stating that both her parents "are diabetic" (line 8), thereby claiming a certain amount of epistemic access. She then expresses her real concern in the form of a short narrative about an experience with her mother (lines 8–9 and 14) in which her blood sugar levels were dangerously low, causing her to go into a diabetic coma. Ms. Piper again demonstrates her epistemic access with relation to diabetes through this story, showing that she knows the dangers of low blood sugar levels. June first aligns with Ms. Piper's narrative experience, even upgrading her evaluative assessment of the situation as "very scary" (line 15). In doing so, June acknowledges Ms. Piper's concerns, possibly in an effort to create rapport with her, even though, as is shown later in the excerpt, low blood sugar levels are not especially concerning for June. June then shifts the topic entirely (line 17) by asking about Ms. Piper's family and work life, topics that do not seem relevant to Ms. Piper's concerns about low blood sugar. This shift indicates a lack of desire to discuss low blood sugars and a lack of concern about this topic.

In the second part of the excerpt, June focuses on the need to get blood sugar levels into a healthy range, a way of enacting her epistemic authority by redirecting the talk to what she sees as most pressing. She explains that Ms. Piper's blood sugar should be in the one hundreds, what she refers to as "good number(s)" (lines 137–138, 144, 148 & 151) and that it is in her "best interest to get out of the big numbers" (lines 159–160) "quickly" (line 153). June draws on her epistemic authority of working with patients with high blood sugars to draw Ms. Piper's attention to what she views as the most significant concern and, in doing so, increases Ms. Piper's knowledge of diabetes to include issues of high blood sugar levels, not just low.

Additionally, June reinforces her epistemic authority through aligning with the patient by acknowledging her symptoms of low blood sugar but prioritizing reliance on empirical data rather than sensations, as they can be an unreliable measure. She cautions Ms. Piper not to rely on feelings of "shaky, sweaty" (line 140) or more generally feeling "crappy" (line 134) but instead, in these moments, to check her blood sugar (lines 134, 141) and use that data instead. June's information sharing in this part is twofold. First, she is foregrounding the information that she knows to be most significant. As she explains to Ms. Piper earlier in the visit, there is "a lot to talk about with diabetes" and that it is "too much" to focus on all of it. Instead, she focuses on what is most significant for Ms. Piper at this moment. Second, by acknowledging Ms. Piper's fears in the first part of the excerpt and referencing the symptoms of low blood sugar in the second part, she is likely trying to alleviate some of her fears by stating that she will "be a lo:ng way from going into a coma" (135, 132). Mooney and Ryan (1993) suggest that patients are often seeking information that can reduce their anxiety about their illness. June's focus on getting patients to rely on empirical data rather than feelings, a topic which is addressed in many of her visits, is likely a way to do this.

At the end of the excerpt, Ms. Piper once again returns to her concern of low blood sugar by asking specifically what these symptoms are, noted by the elongated vowel and rising intonation at the end of the utterance (line 163).[2] Again, June does not allow this topic to continue and states specifically that she will not address that question at this point, announcing the topic she wants to discuss: "we'll get to that later let me tell you about your medicine now" (164–165). June's redirection of the topic as well as her final refusal to answer Ms. Piper's question seems contradictory to the patient-centered approach in that she does not allow the patient to be a co-contributor in determining the content the visit. In fact, prior research on medical visits have viewed these types of topic shifts and the ways in which providers control topics as evidence of the asymmetry in medical visits and the ways in which providers do not allow patients equal access to the floor (c.f. Heritage & Clayman, 2010; Roter & Hall, 1992). Although this may be the case, June is not simply *ignoring* Ms. Piper's topic; she addresses it but only within the larger context of relying on empirical data (i.e. testing her blood sugar) and addressing Ms. Piper's more immediate need of getting her blood sugar levels into the normal range. Redirecting the talk does reflect the asymmetric power dynamic of the visit, but this does not mean that the patient's concern and/or best interest is ignored. Her concern is addressed, albeit not directly but within a larger discussion of feelings associated with lowering her blood sugar levels to a safe and acceptable range. In fact, June's avoidance of directly addressing the question in line 163 is in Ms. Piper's best interest. If, at this point, June described the symptoms of low blood sugar, Ms. Piper might fixate on it, particularly since she has already expressed concerns about it. It is also likely that she is attempting to mitigate Ms. Piper's fears surrounding diabetes by reminding her to trust empirical data rather than feelings or symptoms.

As an NP who specializes in diabetes care, June has greater epistemic authority and access. She relies on her knowledge to determine what to share with patients and when. Although Ms. Piper seems concerned with levels that are dangerously low, June redirects these concerns, first by changing the topic altogether (line 17), backgrounding sensations/symptoms of low blood sugars while prioritizing the need for empirically checking blood sugar levels and relying on that data to determine whether or not the patient is within the healthy range (lines 132–162), and finally by putting the question off to a later time (line 164). In doing so, June gives Ms. Piper greater epistemic access, particularly in relation to focusing on healthy numbers rather than seemingly unhealthy sensations.

3.2   How Does That Happen in Just Two Years?

The next excerpt occurs later in the same visit between June and Ms. Piper. Ms. Piper, in adjusting to her new diagnosis of diabetes, begins this excerpt by explaining that her rise in blood sugar levels was sudden in her view. She then poses the question, "how does that happen in just two years" (line 6), which could be intended as rhetorical but is taken up by June as information-seeking. June then explains how blood sugar levels can change rapidly (lines 5–8), what happens to the body when it stops producing insulin (lines 8–29), and how medical providers are able to accurately diagnose diabetes (lines 32–35). Throughout the excerpt, she uses lay terminology and a low register to make the information more accessible to Ms. Piper, thereby increasing her epistemic access.

Excerpt 2

```
1.  Ms. Piper: because the nurse looked (.) I mean I was in the
2.             hospital two years ago my blood sugar was one
3.             twenty (3.5) it was over four hundred (1.0) when I
4.             got here
5.  June:      okay=
6.  Ms. Piper:       =how does that happen in just two years,
7.  June:      it can happen in two months when the pancreas has
8.             had enough and it cannot produce enough insulin in
9.             the face of all the (.) challenges and ↑ workload (.) it
10.            will start to shut itself down it cannot meet the
11.            challenge anymore (1.0) the pancreas is an organ
12.            over on that side of your ↑ belly [it produces
13. Ms. Piper:                                  [mmhmm
14. June:      several hormones pan- insulin is only one hormone
15.            that it produces but it's the only place we get insulin
16.            (1.0) insulin is the hormone that goes out and grabs
17.            ↑ glucose (.) in the blood stream (.) and grabs ahold of
18.            it and moves it through the (.) body and into the
19.            cell walls it's the only way glucose gets into the cell
20.            when glucose stays in the (.) blood stream (.) in a big
21.            number then they suck water from all the rest of the
22.            body and the blood stream because it's trying to
23.            dilute all those big ↑ molecules so where does all that
```

24.   go:? through the kidney (.) and you pee a lot (1.0)
25.   and because you're peeing a lot your brain says 'I'm
26.   losing water' and it stimulates thirst (1.0) and
27.   because glucose doesn't get in the cells where its
28.   supposed to fuel your ↑ body you (.) pee your food
29.   out into the toilet (.) literally (.) you lose weight, (.)
30.   so the symptoms that you've been having? are high
31.   blood sugar symptoms (0.5) when the blood sugar (.)
32.   in the morning is ↑ high (.) we can diagnose diabetes,
33.   (.) when it's high anytime in a spot check, we can
34.   diagnose diabetes or we can use an A1C which is an
35.   average blood ↑ glucose
36. Ms. Piper: mhm
37. June: and your average is three hundred (.) so we can
38.   diagnose diabetes off of that (.) any way we cut it we
39.   know that you have diabetes, (1.0) and we can fix
40.   that

Even though Ms. Piper's question (in line 6) could be interpreted as a rhetorical question, it indicates her lack of knowledge of how someone gets diabetes. Based on June's description, it is also clear that Ms. Piper's lack of knowledge can explain how she missed the signs of diabetes (i.e. excessive thirst and frequent urination), which she previously acknowledged to have been experiencing for "a couple years." June, presumably, views this as her professional and epistemic responsibility to share what Ms. Piper does not know about her newly diagnosed condition: first, briefly answering her question in lines 7–11, and then, more explicitly in the rest of the excerpt. Understanding her epistemic responsibility to provide Ms. Piper with accessible information, June uses a number of nontechnical lexical choices, namely "belly" (line 12) and "pee"/"peeing" (lines 24, 25, 28) as well as the verbs "grabs" (line 17), "moves" (line 18), and "suck" (line 21) to describe the role that insulin plays. One could argue that June's use of low-register terms such as "belly" and "pee" are more patronizing than helpful; however, as she noted in an interview with me, individuals' cognitive processing as well as ability to retain information is severely reduced during an inpatient stay or after receiving a stressful or emotional diagnosis (also supported by research, c.f. Kessels, 2003); therefore, these terms are likely employed in order to aid Ms. Piper in both processing and retaining the information. Additionally, she intermingles more scientific terms such as "molecules" (line 23) and "glucose" (lines 17, 19, 20, 27, 34), with the low-register terms, giving Ms. Piper greater epistemic access to the technical vocabulary of diabetes. June also lacks specificity in terms of the amount of glucose in the blood that can cause damage, referred to as an unspecified "big number" (lines 20–21) and her informal, nontechnical description of how the brain sends signals to the body through her use of the quotative: "your brain says 'I'm losing water'" (lines 25–26). As Kessels reports, "statements in simple language will be recalled better than complex formulations" (200: 221). June's explanation follows what research such as Kessels' suggests, which is that an effective way of sharing knowledge is through 'simple language.'

June's description of the process specifically addresses previously discussed topics such as Ms. Piper's frequent urination and excessive thirst. In doing so, she relates new information directly to Ms. Piper's experience, addressing their shared knowledge of Ms. Piper's symptoms, which she most directly references in line 30. She acknowledges Ms. Piper's own epistemic access of her experiences and draws on that to provide an explanation and answer to her question of how this could happen in what she sees as a relatively short time span. She uses rising intonation on "having" (line 30), possibly further highlighting their shared knowledge of her previous experiences or "common ground" knowledge (Brazil, 1997). She also uses the rhetorical question "so where does all that go?" in lines 23 and 24, possibly as a way to draw Ms. Piper into this description and focus her attention on the important point, which is to explain why excessive urination is a symptom of untreated diabetes.

At the end of her explanation of how insulin works, June also introduces a term "A1C," which is a test commonly used and commonly referred to in diabetes management. June, relying on her knowledge of Ms. Piper as newly diagnosed, likely defines this term for her as she recognizes an epistemic need for this information. Again, she provides a somewhat simple and nonspecific way of defining A1C rather than giving extraneous information that Ms. Piper likely does not need nor would remember at this point. The description of how diabetes works seems to provide general education to Ms. Piper, based on her own inquiry about how she developed diabetes without realizing it. This information both increases Ms. Piper's access, addressing her right to know about her illness, and likely calms some of her fears (Mooney & Ryan, 1993) simply by providing more information to her regarding not just the treatment but how diabetes effects the body.

3.3 That's Bread, Pasta Sweets That's Carbs

Working in a different context of outpatient primary care, Laura also employs nontechnical language in order to increase a patient's epistemic access. In this excerpt, Laura describes Mr. Barnes' recent blood work to him. Rather than simply reporting the data, she presents it along with the expected norms and 'translates' various aspects of his lipid profile (e.g. triglycerides, LDL, HDL, and total cholesterol) into common food items and categories. Unlike the previous example, Laura does not explain what happens in the body, when, for example, we consume high levels of cholesterol; instead, her approach is to relate the test results to dietary habits. Also, she does not avoid the technical terms; instead, her tactic is to present them alongside the 'translated' food items and dietary choices.

Excerpt 3

1. Laura: your triglycerides are three hundred and thirty-two, (.)
2. they should be below one fifty that's bread pastas
3. sweets that's carbs okay so you need to cut back on that
4. and look at where you were last time you had blood work
5. Mr. Barnes: okay
6. Laura: so from one twenty-six you're up to three hundred and
7. thirty-two so you need to watch yer::: yer diet
8. Mr. Barnes: okay back to what I was doin'
9. Laura: well that's right try not to be eating a lot of sweets or breads
10. Mr. Barnes: okay
11. Laura: all right your LDL which is the bad cholesterol that
12. clogs up the arteries is one seventy-nine, okay it
13. should be below one sixty that's pork products red
14. meats saturated fats [okay::
15. Mr. Barnes: [aw no pork?
16. Laura: so you have to eat more turkey chicken fish,
17. Mr. Barnes: fish okay tuna
18. Laura: a:nd it is better than it was last time you were two
19. hundred 'n two (.) now you're down to one seventy-nine
20. but [you need to be a little lower
21. Mr. Barnes: [need to get it all lower
22. Laura: definitely
23. Mr. Barnes: okay
24. Laura: your cholesterol is two hundred sixty-six it should be

25.   below two hundred,
26. Mr. Barnes: okay [I gotta cut off on my <u>french</u> fries
27. Laura: [so::   well that's right fried foods um:
28.   last time you were at two sixty, (.) so you're a little bit <u>higher</u>
29. Mr. Barnes: okay

In describing each of the components of the lipid panel: triglycerides, HDL, LDL, and total cholesterol, Laura tells Mr. Barnes what his test results are as well as what would be considered healthy (lines 1–2, 11–13 and 25). This is important information for patients to know, particularly when their readings are far above what is considered acceptable, as is the case with Mr. Barnes' triglycerides and total cholesterol levels. Although she does not provide specific feedback in how to improve these numbers, she does 'translate' each aspect of the lipid panel into the food sources that contribute to each. In lines 2–3, for example, she translates triglycerides into "breads pastas sweets…carbs"; similarly, LDL is translated into avoidance of "pork products red meats" (lines 13–14) and increased consumption of "turkey chicken fish" (line 16). The patients' uptake of this approach and translation technique seems to be fairly effective. First, he reports back the information: "no pork?" (line 15) and "fish okay tuna" (line 17). By the third example, he initiates his own translation of health data to food in line 26, where he interprets his high total cholesterol into "I gotta cut off on my <u>french</u> fries," which the NP confirms in the following line "that's right fried foods" (line 27), recasting the information and aligning with his prior turn. Through the repeated process of providing (1) the technical term, (2) Mr. Barnes' readings, (3) the healthy range, and (4) the translation into dietary choices, Laura increases Mr. Barnes' epistemic access. She provides information that he needs in order to improve his health, focusing on simple choices, made accessible through her use of clear, simplified dietary changes or substitutions.

In addition to translating the information for Mr. Barnes into easily comprehended data, Laura also includes Mr. Barnes in her reading and interpretation of his medical tests. This occurs in lines 4–7. In line 4, after discussing Mr. Barnes' triglyceride reading, she draws the patient into the discussion and into her task of reading and interpreting the data through the directive: "look at where you were last time." Although audio recordings cannot confirm that she physically shows the data to Mr. Barnes, the use of the directive here suggests that she does, in fact, show him the data to reinforce the difference between his previous reading ("last time") and his current reading, which indicates a significant increase and one that took him out of the acceptable and healthy range. Here, Laura seems to be addressing the dimension of epistemic primacy, in her awareness of Mr. Barnes' right to direct access to specific information about his health rather than it exclusively being transmitted through her.

3.4 I Don't Tell Too Many People This

The last excerpt in this chapter also involves June and another patient who has been hospitalized with high blood sugar levels. The patient, Mr. Tucker, is not newly diagnosed with diabetes but is finding that his occupational requirements and the medication he is currently on are not enough for him. Throughout the visit, June and Mr. Tucker discuss ways that he can deal with these complications, including being on insulin for as long as possible. Just before the excerpt, June has explained this to him. The excerpt starts with Mr. Tucker repeating that information (line 1) and June providing greater detail about why this is the case. Similar to excerpt 2 with Ms. Piper, June explains important information about diabetes, this time focusing on the positive repercussions of lowering the A1C. Because Mr. Tucker displays a higher level of knowledge about diabetes than Ms. Piper, June uses more technical information and goes into greater detail with him.

Excerpt 4

1. Mr. Tucker: and the longer I can keep it down (.) [the better (.)
2. June: [yeah the
3. Mr. Tucker: numbers'll [get
4. June: [yes YES 'cuz there's a thing called
5.   glucose <u>toxicity</u> that says the ↑ higher that A1C is?
6.   (1.0) the harder it is for your (.) medicines to do its
7.   job so more <u>days</u> and more <u>weeks</u> on ↑ insulin
8.   getting the numbers fixed gettin' the A1C down?
9.   (1.0) means your <u>pills</u> can be a little more powerful
10.   and A1C is that <u>average</u> its made up of three to four
11.   months average glucose (1.0) because that
12.   hemoglobin A:: is <u>stuck</u> to the side of the red blood
13.   cell and thats what acts like a sponge

... *(6 lines omitted)*
19. June: actually I don't tell too many people this 'cuz they're not
20.   too interested in the numbers but each drop of an
21.   A1C (1.0) each <u>percent</u> (.) and you've gone down
22.   <u>three</u>, (.) decreases your risk of amputation fourteen
23.   percent so fourteen times three (1.0) it decreases
24.   your risk of <u>stroke</u> (.) like ↑ seven percent so each
25.   percent A1C is a <u>really</u> big deal so when you tell me
26.   you've gone from fifteen to ↑ twelve I know what that
27.   means (.) I get it (.) I know what that means that's (1.0)
28.   big and if you can go from twelve to ten (1.5) that's super
29.   big (1.0) so the A1C turns over when the red blood
30.   cells turn ↑ <u>over</u> that's what we're measuring red blood
31.   cells that've been exposed to ↑ glucose (1.0) and if we
32.   ha- we say it's a three to four month average the scientists
33.   tell me that the <u>last</u> ↑ month of blood sugar control (.)
34.   weighs a little bit heavier than others (.0 so (.) so even a
35.   few <u>weeks</u> of insulin, (.) would have a greater effect

Prior to this exchange, Mr. Tucker has shown that he has a fairly good understanding of his disease. He references the medicine he currently takes and the dosage amounts, showing a level of agency and personal responsibility in his diabetes management. He also references a type of insulin by its brand name, Lantus, when June discusses his need to switch to insulin, showing that he not only knows his medication but is knowledgeable enough about diabetes management to know other medications by name. He has also shared that his previous A1C was three points higher than it is currently. By providing this information, Mr. Tucker illustrates that he (1) knows what A1C is; (2) knows both his current and former readings; and (3) has taken steps to lower his blood sugar levels over the past few months. In fact, June references this information in lines 21 and 22 ("you've gone down three") and displays affiliation with him, "I know what that means I get it," lines 26–27) and acknowledging the efforts he has made ("that's super big," lines 28–29).

June evaluates Mr. Tucker's epistemic access based on what he has shared with her during the visit and addresses his epistemic primacy by providing more technical information than she might otherwise. This is evident in a number of places in the extract. First, June uses higher register, more technical terms including "glucose toxicity" (line 5) and "hemoglobin A" (line 12). She still uses low-register terms like "stuck" (line 12) and compares the process to "a sponge" (line 13), similar to how she describes the process to Ms. Piper, illustrating that she still is making information accessible to Mr. Tucker while expanding his epistemic access by introducing likely new terms (i.e. glucose toxicity) and more technical terminology (i.e. hemoglobin A).

June also orients to Mr. Tucker's level of epistemic access and likely desire to know more in lines 19 and 20, when she states, "actually I don't tell too many people this cuz they're not too interested in the numbers." The initial turn "actually" implies an introduction of novel or surprising information (Aijmer, 2013), suggesting that either June is surprised to be sharing this information or hinting to Mr. Tucker that he is atypical in both his prior knowledge and interest in knowing more. In prefacing the information in this way, June is orienting to what she sees as Mr. Tucker's interest "in the numbers" and is positioning him as not like most people she sees in the hospital. She draws on her own epistemic authority to expand his epistemic access by making reference to the research describing the health benefits of lowering one's A1C (lines 22–24) and the ways in which each month may not be weighed equally (lines 32–34). When comparing this exchange to the one with Ms. Piper, it is clear that June makes the effort to meet her patients where they are in terms of their current level of knowledge while seeking to increase it as a way of providing quality health care.

4 Conclusion

In this chapter, I draw on the 'dimensions of knowledge' framework as put forth by Stivers, Mondada, and Steensig (2011). Although this model requires some modification for it to be applicable to the institutional setting of medical visits, this framework allows/clarifies the NP's choices in terms of what knowledge to share and in what form. Viewing knowledge sharing in terms of NP's epistemic responsibility to "attend not only to who knows what, but also to who has a *right* to know what, who knows *more* about what and who is *responsible* for knowing what" (Stivers et al., 2011, p. 18), NPs prioritize patient's epistemic primacy, or the "right to know what" rather than focusing on what they might already know. This is not to say that the patient's current level of knowledge is not considered. In the case of June working with individuals with diabetes, she tailors the knowledge she shares, based on how much they already know. Ms. Piper shows very little knowledge about her own diabetes, first by worrying about blood sugar levels that are too low rather than her current levels that are too high (excerpt 1) and by lack of knowledge of what diabetes really is and how it develops (excerpt 2). When Mr. Tucker displays a great deal of knowledge about his diabetes and interest in learning more, June ups the ante, if you will, providing more technical and detailed information to him. By comparing these two interactions, it is clear that June does attend to the patients' current level of access in some way, albeit differently than the ways that Stivers et al. (2011) describe for everyday interactions. That is, she does this not by directly asking but by considering their current state (newly diagnosed vs. living with diabetes for a number of years) as well as responding to their interactional displays of knowledge.

There are many reasons that NPs may not overtly ask about patients' current epistemic access. In the case of inpatient visits, this is likely done because of the reduced cognitive processing abilities of individuals who have been hospitalized (Kessels, 2003). In outpatient visits, such as the one between Laura and Mr. Barnes, in which each visit has a predetermined time limit of 30 minutes, NPs need to ensure that patients receive the most significant information for them at that moment. Simply telling them the information is less time-consuming that attempting to determine if they already have that information. Additionally, information-seeking on the part of the NPs could be face-threatening for the patients. For example, if Laura asked Mr. Barnes if he knew what triglycerides were or what foods were associated with them, he would likely feel as though he is being tested and evaluated on his current level of knowledge. Since NPs are in the higher position of authority and have epistemic authority, asking questions, in this case, would likely reinforce the asymmetrical position of the NP and patient rather than diminishing it. Therefore, instead of focusing on determining patients' prior access, these excerpts can be understood in terms of NPs prioritizing patients' primacy or their 'right to know' specific medical information that is relevant to their current condition and needs.

Although this chapter mainly includes examples from June's inpatient visits, the patterns of patient education are evident throughout other visits as well. The example involving Laura and Mr. Barnes illustrates Laura's commitment to educating patients by making information accessible. In an interview with the researcher, Laura described her role as an NP as a 'teacher.' Other NPs in this study use similar terms including 'educator' and 'guide' as a way to describe their role in providing information to patients. The focus on educating patients and knowledge sharing is well documented in the research in terms of the positive health outcomes (Mazzuca et al., 1983; Orth et al., 1987). Moreover, as researchers have noted, most patients are seeking information rather than simply a cure when they visit a health provider (Mooney & Ryan, 1993).

This chapter has outlined some of the forms that knowledge sharing takes in medical visits between NPs and patients. This primarily includes making information accessible to patients through the use of nontechnical terms or avoidance of "medicalese" (Roter & Hall, 1992, p. 93). Other linguistic features include the use of rhetorical questions (excerpt 2), which engage the patient and bring her in as a more active participant rather than a passive recipient of knowledge, recasting the patient's claim of knowledge (except 3), and providing more specific and specialized knowledge when a patient shows interest (excerpt 4). Each of these features can be understood as an enactment of the NPs' epistemic and professional responsibility, that is, the responsibility to make information accessible to patients so that they may empower them to take a greater role in their own health care.

Notes

1. Heath (1992) points out that patients also bring certain information to the visit—namely, knowledge of their symptoms that providers rely on to make an accurate diagnosis. However, the patient's knowledge is understood as being limited compared with that of the provider.
2. It is interesting that June has actually described the symptoms of low blood sugar to Ms. Piper, albeit within the discussion of avoiding high levels and relying on empirical checks, but Ms. Piper does not recognize that information. This seems to support the argument by Kessels (2003) and June herself that patients cannot take in an unlimited amount of information in an acute setting such as this, further supporting June's choice to focus on highs rather than lows.

References

Aijmer, K. (2013). *English discourse particles: Evidence from a corpus*. Amsterdam: John Benjamins.

Beck, R. S., Daughtridge, R., & Sloane, P. D. (2002). Physician-patient communication in the primary care office: A systematic review. *The Journal of the American Board of Family Practice, 15*(1), 25–38.

Brazil, D. (1997). *The communicative value of intonation in English* (2nd ed.). Cambridge: Cambridge University Press.

Charles, C., Gafni, A., & Whelan, T. (1997). Shared decision-making in the medical encounter: What does it mean? (Or it takes at least two to tango). *Social Science & Medicine, 44*(5), 681–692.

Frankel, R. M., & Stein, T. (1999). Getting the most out of the clinical encounter: The four habits model. *The Permanente Journal, 3*(3), 79–88.

Hadlow, J., & Pitts, M. (1991). The understanding of common health terms by doctors, nurses and patients. *Social Science & Medicine, 32*(2), 193–196.

Haidet, P., & Paterniti, D. A. (2003). Building' a history rather than 'taking' one: A perspective on information sharing during the medical interview. *Archives of Internal Medicine, 163*, 1134–1140.

Heath, C. (1992). The delivery and reception of diagnosis and assessment in the general practice consultation. In P. Drew & J. Heritage (Eds.), *Talk at work*. Cambridge: Cambridge University Press.

Heritage, J. (2005). Revisiting authority in physician-patient interaction. In J. Duchan & D. Kovarsky (Eds.), *Diagnosis as cultural practice* (pp. 83–102). New York: Mouton de Gruyter.

Heritage, J., & Clayman, S. (2010). *Talk in action: Interactions, identities, and institutions*. Oxford: Wiley-Blackwell.

Holzner, B. (1968). *Reality construction in society*. Cambridge: Schenkman.

Kessels, R. (2003). Patients' memory for medical information. *Journal of the Royal Society of Medicine, 96*(5), 219–222.

Mazzuca, S. A., Weinberger, M., Kurpius, D. J., Froehle, T. C., & Heister, M. (1983). Clinician communication associated with diabetic patients' comprehension of their therapeutic regimen. *Diabetes Care, 6*, 347–350.

Mishler, E. (1984). *The discourse of medicine: Dialectics of medical interviews*. Norwood, NJ: Ablex.

Mooney, G., & Ryan, M. (1993). Agency in health care: Getting beyond first principles. *Journal of Health Economics, 12*, 125–135.

Orth, J. E., Stiles, W. B., Scherwitz, L., Hennrikus, D., & Vallbona, C. (1987). Patient exposition and provider explanation in routine interviews and hypertensive patient's blood pressure control. *Health Psychology, 6*, 29–42.

Peräkylä, A. (1998). Authority and accountability: The delivery of diagnosis in primary health care. *Social Psychology Quarterly, 61*(4), 301–320.

Roter, D., & Hall, J. (1992/2006). *Doctors talking with patients/patients talking with doctors: Improving communication in medical visits* (2nd ed.). Westport, CT: Praeger.

Stivers, T., Mondada, L., & Steensig, J. (2011). Knowledge, morality and affiliation in social interaction. In T. Stivers, L. Mondada, & J. Steensig (Eds.), *The morality of knowledge in conversation* (pp. 3–26). Cambridge: Cambridge University Press.

Waitzkin, H. (1985). Information giving in medical care. *Journal of Health and Social Behavior, 26*(2), 81–101.

CHAPTER 4

Treading Lightly: Indirect Speech in Medical Directives

Abstract Medical advice and directives are key components of medical care. This chapter addresses how nurse practitioners (NPs) use indirectness to soften the force of medical advice/directives. This is accomplished by using on-record indirectness, in which advice is given with hedges and mitigation, and off-record indirectness, in which advice is hinted at rather than stated outright, and a combination of these tactics. In many cases, indirectness serves a dual purpose of both giving directives and critiquing past behavior; therefore, there is more at stake in terms of threatening the face of the patients. NPs likely employ indirectness strategies in order to avoid these potential face threats and seemingly offer optionality in terms of whether patients must follow the advice, both of which help establish positive relationships with patients.

Keywords Medical advice • Medical critiques • Bivalence • Hedging • Indirectness • Relational work

1 INTRODUCTION

Because providers occupy a position of authority and are expected to deliver clear, unambiguous medical advice, one might expect direct—or at least, on record—strategies in giving medical advice or directives.

However, directives are inherently face threatening for the addressee (Leech, 2014), suggesting a need for more tactful, indirect language. Further complicating this issue is the fact that advice for future behavior often also implicitly entails critique of past behavior, particularly when dealing with long-term chronic illnesses that require a certain amount of personal agency and self-directed care. In this chapter, I argue that one of the ways that nurse practitioners (NPs) enact their professional competency is by couching their directives (and when applicable, critiques) in indirect speech. I explore a number of indirect strategies that NPs employ, including the use of on-record indirectness that is mitigated through hedging and off-record strategies that hint at the advice rather than stating it outright. The reasons for choosing indirectness can likely be attributed to the NPs' patient-centered approach. Indirectness creates a sense of optionality, giving respect to patient's autonomy in decision making and encourages the development of positive provider–patient relationships through a lowered sense of imposition on the patient and a lowering of hierarchical power (Leech, 2014) between provider and patient.

2   Defining Indirect Speech/Indirectness

Indirect speech can reference a variety of linguistic forms, depending on the definition and scope one chooses to apply (c.f. Haugh, 2015 for a comprehensive account of definitions of indirect speech). The earliest definition comes from Searle who defined an indirect speech act (ISA) as a "sentence that contains the illocutionary force indicators for one kind of illocutionary act" but performs, "*in addition*, another type of illocutionary act" (1975, p. 268). That is, an ISA contains essentially two illocutionary acts, or speech acts: the one that is literally uttered and the one that the speaker implicates but does not state outright. An often used example in English is, "Can you close the window?" which has the literal force of a question of the addressee's ability to perform such action, but 'what is implicated' is a directive, a speech act that is associated with imperative forms such as "close the window."[1] Scholarly understanding of indirectness has expanded since Searle's early account, but the notion of the speech act is still relevant in that it acknowledges that there is often (although not always) a 'direct' alternative and that 'what is said' often carries an additional, and even more important, meaning in 'what is implicated.'

Since Searle, researchers have continued to explore the linguistic notion of indirectness, often expanding this original formulation in a number of important ways. First, Searle considered a speech act to be inherent in a single utterance, which neglects to consider how utterances may work together in a particular exchange. That is, "indirectness is not simply a property of individual utterances, but rather can be attributed more holistically to a sequence of utterances" (Haugh, 2015, p. 32). In fact, it may be the case that the full effect or force of indirect speech comes from the cumulative effect of a series of turns rather than residing within an individual utterance. Another point to consider in defining indirectness, and one that is relevant to this chapter, is the fact that utterances may have more than one indirect meaning. Jenny Thomas (1986) employs the terms 'bivalent' and 'plurivalent' to address these multiple intended meanings. Thomas suggests that, rather than a single implicature, a speaker may intend to communicate two (i.e. bivalent) or more (i.e. plurivalent) messages. She gives the example of a mother uttering the following: "Are those your filthy socks decorating the bathroom floor?" (1986, p. 163) as having the indirect meaning of both scolding the child for leaving his/her socks on the floor and giving a directive to the child to pick the socks up. These multiple layers of meaning are integral to understanding the examples of indirectness presented in this chapter, as many of them can be interpreted as 'bivalent' in that the NPs seem to be simultaneously critiquing past behavior as well as giving medical directives for future behavior.

Indirectness can also be understood in terms not just of *what* is said but *how* it is said. Lempert (2012), for example, uses the term "indirect addressivity," which, rather than focusing on the linguistic form, considers the literal and/or intended addressee (see also Kiesling and Johnson's (2010) discussion of production indirection). For example, an addressee may not be directly addressed; instead, the intended addressee must recognize that the message is for him/her. Morgan (1991) provides a similar discussion of indirectness in her work on African American women's discourse. She argues that within this community two types of indirectness are common: pointed and baited. Pointed indirectness is similar to indirect addressivity in that it involves a "sham receiver" (420, citing Fisher, 1976), or an addressee who is not the intended audience. Baited indirectness requires similar work on the part of the addressee to recognize that she is the intended audience since she is not being directly addressed. Tannen (2010) employs the term "ventriloquizing" to describe another type of indirectness in which a speaker temporarily takes on the voice of another as a way to distance the speaker (rather than the addressee) from the message. In this way, ventriloquizing is not indirect in terms of what is said per se, but how it is said. Although not a comprehensive account of how indirect speech can be defined, these more recent definitions, along with Searle's account of the ISA, provide a framework for understanding the excerpts presented in this chapter.

2.1 Forms of Indirectness

One way of conceiving of indirectness is to consider levels or degrees of indirectness. An important distinction in this respect is the difference between on-record and off-record indirectness. A distinction proposed by Brown and Levinson (1987), on-record indirectness involves references to the intended speech act, but presented in some mitigated way. The example provided earlier, of "Can you close the window?" would be an example of on-record indirectness. The directive is mitigated through the use of the interrogative form, as opposed to an imperative, but it still makes reference to the desired action ('closing the window'), the object of the request ('the window), and the intended actor/addressee ('you'). On-record indirectness may also involve mitigation strategies. Mitigation strategies such as hedges give the impression of reducing "responsibility and obligations" (Thaler, 2012, p. 909) or can reduce the intensity of an implicature and "thereby further the achievement of interactional goals" (Caffi, 1999, p. 882). For example, "Could you close that window just a bit?" with the addition of "just a bit" is still on-record for the same reasons discussed above, but with the impression of the action being smaller and less imposing on the hearer. On-record strategies still lessen the severity or the degree of imposition of the intended speech act but likely do not impede interpretation on the part of the hearer. Off-record indirectness, on the other hand, involves utterances in which "there is more than one unambiguously attributable intention so that the actor cannot be held to have committed himself [sic] to a particular intent" (Brown & Levinson, 1987, p. 69). Off-record indirectness can give both the speaker and the hearer an 'out' by either claiming to not have intended the implicated meaning or not having interpreted the indirectness implied. An example of off-record indirectness might involve a declarative such as "it's a bit cold in here," in which the request for the window to be closed is veiled as a statement of the condition of the room without mention of either the request (i.e. to close) or the object in question (i.e. the window). In the case of off-record indirectness, the hearer is required to do a greater amount of interpretive work to infer the speaker's intended meaning. Leech refers to these as hints or "hinting strategies" (2014, p. 142). In the data presented in this chapter, both on-record and off-record strategies are employed when giving medical directives.

2.2   Explanations for Indirectness

The most common explanation for a speaker to choose an indirect strategy is tied to the concept of face, or one's public self-image (Goffman, 1967). Brown and Levinson (1987) propose that indirect speech is a politeness tactic that can be understood in terms of attending to the face of either the speaker or the hearer by avoiding face-threatening acts (FTA). Face, according to Brown and Levinson, comprises both "positive face" (the desire to be approved of by others) and "negative face" (the desire for autonomy in one's actions). Various speech acts are associated with a hearer's positive face and negative face; directives, for example, impede on one's desire for autonomy, or negative face, while critiques are associated with one's positive face, or desire for approval. Schneider takes a somewhat wider view of indirect speech. Primarily focusing on mitigation devices, he argues that mitigation constructs a type of relational work, which includes Brown and Levinson's concept of facework as well as other interpersonal goals. Schneider defines relational work as "the linguistic activities carried out by interactants when they negotiate relationships with one another and adapt their own language to different speech events and different goals" (2010, p. 254). He argues that the use of mitigation "facilitates the management of interpersonal relations" by achieving a "compromise between what the speaker wants to say and what the interlocutor is willing to accept" (2010, p. 255). Within the clinical setting, mitigated or even more indirect forms of medical advice may allow a compromise between inherently face-threatening directives and the desire to maintain positive relationships.

2.3   Indirectness in Medical Visits

As noted in the introduction, directives in medical care pose an interesting social and clinical problem. On the one hand, as Bonnefon, Feeney and DeNeys point out, medical encounters involve high stakes, which seem to warrant directness and clarity, so as to avoid leaving "one in a greater state of uncertainty about what is really meant" (2011, p. 322). That is, choosing a more direct strategy means that a provider's message is more likely to be interpreted as intended. Additionally, considering the asymmetric dynamic of medical visits in which the provider is not only in a position to provide directives and/or instructions, but also in a position in which the patient is actively soliciting aid and advice from his/her provider, it may seem unnecessary to give advice in a mitigated, indirect manner. However, from a social perspective, directives (and other related speech acts such as advice, orders, and instructions) threaten the hearer's negative face, or the right act autonomously and unimpeded. This seems to leave medical providers in a complicated predicament as to how to deliver medical advice. As other researchers have noted, despite the high-stakes nature and the inherent power imbalance of medical encounters, indirectness is used quite frequently in medical visits across a range of provider types (Benkendorf, Prince, Rose, De Fina, & Hamilton, 2001: genetic counselors; Caffi, 1999: psychotherapists; Defibaugh, 2014: nurse practitioners; Parry, 2005: physiotherapists). Parry (2005), for instance, notes that despite being specifically trained to be direct, the physiotherapists in her study often use mitigation tactics, particularly hedges, when discussing something problematic about the patient's health or progress. Benkendorf and colleagues, in their study of genetic counselors, posit that "the use of indirect speech may be underpinned by the professional mandate to be nondirective and client-centered" (2001, p. 206) suggesting that genetic counselors equate nondirective counseling with indirect language. NPs, although not engaged in nondirective care, are focused on providing patient-centered care, which may explain the use of indirect strategies to give medical directives. The desire for indirectness is likely even stronger when there is the additional implicit criticism involved. NPs can provide a couched criticism of past, unhealthy behavior within an indirect medical directive, thereby doing double duty in terms of interpersonal work by minimizing threats to the patient's positive face by avoiding direct criticism as well as minimizing threats to his/her negative face by mitigating the force of the directive.

3 MEDICAL ADVICE, CRITIQUES, AND INDIRECT SPEECH

The following excerpts each present a slightly different way in which medical advice is given, focusing on how the NPs use indirectness to varying degrees and how this correlates with the additional speech act of offering criticisms. Starting with examples that are seemingly direct, excerpts 1 and 2, reveal how even direct imperatives can be understood as being indirect in some way, either by lacking in specificity of the advice (excerpt 1) or by implicating an additional directive with a single imperative (excerpt 2). The last three excerpts illustrate how indirectness can be used to simultaneously provide advice for future behavior while also critiquing past behavior. In each of these excerpts, the indirectness takes a different form: excerpt 3 shows how Laura's use of mitigation and hedging over multiple turns softens the force of the implicature in a way that an individual turn could not; in excerpt 4, Julie uses off-record indirectness through a medical explanation that only hints at the advice and critique; finally, excerpt 5 illustrates how June uses multiple indirect strategies, including indirect addressivity (Lempert, 2012). In each of these cases, indirectness can be understood in terms of the NPs engaging in 'relational work' by avoiding potential face threats, creating opportunities for treatment to be negotiated through seeming optionality, and the construction of positive provider–patient relationships.

3.1 *Concentrate Your Efforts*

The following is the most direct of the exchanges presented in this chapter, at least on the surface. It comes from an inpatient visit between June and Mr. Bray. Mr. Bray has been diagnosed with type 2 diabetes during his current hospitalization and is struggling with knowing how to deal with high and low blood sugars as well as how often to check his blood sugar. Earlier in this exchange, he tells June that he is "anal" and wonders if he should check his blood sugar frequently and take corrective measures. June then goes on to explain the process of blood sugars changing throughout the day and the problem of "too much data" which can lead to over-correcting. In the excerpt below, she mimics his use of the term "anal" and praises his desire to be vigilant of his newly diagnosed disease, but then provides seemingly direct advice (lines 1–2); however, the specific details of the medical directive come later (lines 3–5), outside of the imperative.

Excerpt 1

1. June: when you say you're anal about this that's really good but
2. concentrate your efforts where its gonna give you the most
3. bang for your buck and that is about judiciously checking
4. four times a day eating the right amount of carbohydrates taking

5.   the doses on time and referring to the book for decision making
6. Mr. Bray: its more the trouble shooting for a lack of a better word
7. June: right

In this excerpt, June uses the imperative form for the advice "concentrate your efforts" (lines 1–2) but then follows this up by providing more specific advice (lines 3–5). Although June offers the direct imperative of "concentrate your efforts," it is vague in terms of actual medical advice. Instead, this information comes later in June's utterance in the form of a prepositional phase and series of gerundive noun phrases: "checking," "eating," "taking," and "referring." The use of the direct advice seems to function as a way of getting Mr. Bray's attention and connecting her advice back to the previous discussion of him wanting to check too frequently. The actual advice of what Mr. Bray should do: check his blood sugar four times a day, eat the right amount of carbohydrates, take the doses on time, and refer to the book for decision making is not actually part of the imperative structure; it is separate from it, in its own clause and within a prepositional phrase. In this way, the bold, on-record directive does not actually contain the medical advice. In this exchange, June uses a combination of directness to present vague, nonspecific advice, but follows this up with a more indirect form of the specific advice she wants Mr. Bray to follow, creating a kind of softening or distancing effect, minimizing the force of the advice.

3.2   Buy It over the Counter

The second excerpt also seems, at first glance, to only contain a direct imperative, but the imperative has an additional meaning beyond what is said. In this excerpt, the NP, Karen, tells Mr. Eggers that he needs to buy a vitamin supplement (line 11); however, looking at the larger exchange, it is clear that this imperative is referencing both a direct speech act: "buy the medicine over the counter" and an ISA: "take the medication."

Excerpt 2

1. Karen: ah your blood work (.) are you taking the vitamin d over
2.   the counter
3. Mr Eggers: no but I have to start now
4. Karen: okay
5. Mr Eggers: in the summer time I'm outside in the summer time all the
6.   time
7. Karen: right

8. Mr Eggers: and I I think that might- actually
9. Karen: so you weren't taking it
10. Mr Eggers: I I was not taking it
11. Karen: that's okay so vitamin d three buy it over the counter its
12. cheaper two thousand units a day okay
13. Mr Eggers: mhm
14. Karen: make sure you buy that cuz your normal-
15. Mr Eggers: I'm gonna make sure ##
16. Karen: normal is um from thirty to a hundred and yours is twenty-
17. seven okay

In this exchange, Karen first inquires as to whether or not Mr. Eggers is currently taking vitamin D (line 1). Mr. Eggers responds that he is not but, without further prompting from Karen, claims that he needs "to start now." Karen clarifies (line 9) that Mr. Eggers had not previously been taking it and then uses the imperative not to state that he does, in fact, need to start taking it, but to direct him how to acquire the medication, "buy it over the counter it's cheaper" (line 11). On the surface, this direct imperative looks just like that—a direct command of where to buy the medication based on the cost. However, taken with the prior discussion which confirmed that Mr. Eggers had not previously been taking this medication indicates that Karen, in addition, is giving the medical advice to start this medication. This interpretation is further supported by her use of the imperative again in line 14, "make sure you buy that," which this time is followed by an explanation of his vitamin D levels (lines 14 and 16–17). An explanation of the vitamin D levels does not actually provide justification for why he needs to "buy it over the counter" but instead reinforces the point that it is important for him to take the medication. In this excerpt, the imperatives of "buy it over the counter" and "make sure you buy that" serve a dual function of both directing Mr. Eggers to the most cost-effective way of purchasing the vitamin D but also as a way of giving the directive to start taking the supplement.

The following three excerpts represent a slightly different use of indirectness in that they involve both advice-giving and critique, what Thomas (1986) refers to as "bivalent."

3.3 *Every Now and Then You Have to Go See a Urologist*

In the following excerpt, Laura, the NP, and Mr. Vaughn are discussing his current health screening. Through this, she discovers that he has stopped his annual appointments with the urologist. In the excerpt, she is both subtly and indirectly critiquing his past behavior of stopping these annual visits as well as advising him to make an appointment and start going again. She does this through the use of extensive mitigation. Mitigation, as Caffi (1999) shows, is an important tool in discourse likely because it works to achieve an interactional goal. In this example, Laura uses on-record, mitigated advice to both minimize the extent to which she positions herself as a figure of authority and to minimize the 'cost' of the advice to the patient, that is, how much effort it will require on his part.

Excerpt 3

1. Laura: we::ll that's hematuria micro hematuria microscopic
2. blood cells in the urine and I think (.) ((mouse clicking))
3. did you ah:: see a urologist are you still going to see
4. [your urologist?
5. Mr. Vaughn: [no I haven't saw him for some time but yeah (.) it
6. (0.5) other words uh kinda like blood in the urine
7. right? [Or not
8. Laura: [yeah blood in the urine right
9. Mr. Vaughn: yeh well he told me all the time ya know it was probly
10. from scar tissue from my surgery
11. Laura: scar tissue from your surgery?=
12. Mr. Vaughn: =yeah=
13. Laura: =okay
14. Mr. Vaughn: cuz I had my prostrate removed
15. Laura: okay all [right
16. Mr. Vaughn: [yeah that's what he told me all the time
17. Laura: okay (.) s- so generally after you have:: (1.0) ya know
18. prostate cancer ↑ and surgery::
19. Mr. Vaughn: yeah
20. Laura: every now and then you have to go see the uro:logist (.) so
21. Mr. Vaughn: yeah I should go see him [again probably
22. Laura: [yeah yeah because it's
23. surveillance
24. Mr. Vaughn: yeah
25. Laura: its surveillance to make sure that everything is [okay
26. Mr. Vaughn: [yeah yeah
27. Laura: and I did make a copy: two more copies of your blood
28. work for your doctors so share that with [them
29. Mr. Vaughn: [okay

30. Laura: and one for [you
31. Mr. Vaughn: [okay
32. Laura: but um ya know with a history of prostate cancer you
33. need to have surveillance
34. Mr. Vaughn: yeah
35. Laura: just to make sure [that everything is okay
36. Mr. Vaughn: [well that's what I could never figure
37. out I was going to him all the time going to him
38. after I had the surgery (.) and well he said 'yeah you
39. should come back' you know I guess the cancer ↑ could
40. come back or something=
41. Laura: =well that's right (.) cuz what
42. needs to happen (.) ya know until ya leave this earth,
43. ya know a PSA needs to be (.) done
44. Mr. Vaughn: oh yeah okay
45. Laura: ya know blood tests
46. Mr. Vaughn: okay
47. Laura: now your PSA came back fine::, it's less than zero point
48. zero one which [is
49. Mr. Vaughn: [oh that's good yeah
50. Laura: good we get concerned once its one point zero
51. Mr. Vaughn: oh
52. Laura: if it's going ↑ up (.)
53. Mr. Vaughn: [oh yeah
54. Laura: [then something else is going on=
55. Mr. Vaughn: =you read articles
56. though where they say that PSA is [yeah
57. Laura: [yeah
58. Mr. Vaughn: maybe maybe hhh
59. Laura: yeah well I-
60. Mr. Vaughn: but you still think it's a good idea=
61. Laura: =oh I think it's a good idea
62. Mr. Vaughn: I'll probly make an appointment with [them
63. Laura: [yeah I- I think it's
64. a good idea
65. Mr. Vaughn: cuz I haven't been to 'em in probably four or five years
66. time goes by so Fast you know
67. Laura: well I- just to kinda touch base
68. Mr. Vaughn: yeah
69. Laura: just to touch base (.) be<u>cause</u> ya still have blood in the ↑
70. urine
71. Mr. Vaughn: yeah

72. Laura: just to make sure tha:t ya know nothing else is going on
73. Mr. Vaughn: yeah
74. Laura: ya know blood in the urine yes could be from scar tissue::
75. [but it can also be
76. Mr. Vaughn: [yeah
77. Laura: from bladder cancer
78. Mr. Vaughn: okay
79. Laura: okay
80. Mr. Vaughn: yeah
81. Laura: so sometimes if you have microscopic blood in the urine
82. ah: (.) and you've had it for years and you've had it
83. worked up its its just ya know part of your medical history
84. Mr. Vaughn: yeah
85. Laura: but [because of your-
86. Mr. Vaughn: [it's a possibility it could be something else=
87. Laura: =well that's
88. right because of your history of (.) prostate cancer [okay?
89. Mr. Vaughn: [oh yeah
90. Laura: so you want to be sure ah touch base with a
91. urologist [okay?
92. Mr. Vaughn: [yeah yeah okay
93. (1.0) I should I should get a copy of and to take to
94. [him?
95. Laura: [yeah yeah you're gonna ge- go home with two
96. Mr. Vaughn: okay
97. Laura: one for him and one for your private doctor
98. Mr. Vaughn: oh yeah okay

In this exchange between Laura and Mr. Vaughn, there are a number of turns that can be interpreted as giving medical advice. The excerpt begins when Laura asks Mr. Vaughn if he is still going to see a urologist. Since Laura has Mr. Vaughn's medical history accessible on her computer, it is likely that she already knows the answer to this question. Therefore, this question functions as a pre-sequence (Levinson, 1983), or more specifically as pre-advice, essentially 'testing the waters' to determine whether advice is necessary. After indicating that he previously visited the urologist on a regular basis, Mr. Vaughn then acknowledges that he has not gone "for some time" (line 5). This opens the floor for Laura to offer medical advice in lines 17–20. Although Laura uses a conventionalized form of advice in "you have to" (line 20), the advice is prefaced with multiple mitigating devices, lessening the strength of the advice. For example, the use of "generally" (line 17) distances the patient from the advice, making it seem to apply to anyone in this situation rather than just him. "Generally" also has the effect of changing the interpretation of 'you' to be inclusive—again referencing 'anyone' rather than the patient alone. Another mitigation tool is the lack of specificity implicated in the use of "every now and then" (line 20) in reference to the frequency of the visits, giving the effect of less frequent than what is actually required, which is annually (American Society for Clinical Oncology, 2017). It also creates as sense of a somewhat low-ranked imposition on the patient, suggesting that the 'cost' to him is minimal.

First appearing in line 17 but recurrent in Laura's advice-giving throughout (lines 17, 32, 42, 43, 45, 72 and 74) is the discourse marker "ya know," which Schiffrin (1988) refers to as a marker of 'meta-knowledge' shared by speaker and hearer or by the general population. These uses of "ya know" throughout have the effect of mitigating the force of the advice by suggesting that this is knowledge the hearer likely already has but is simply being reminded of. In this respect, it can also be seen as lowering what Leech (2014) refers to as vertical distance (Brown and Levinson (1987) use the term 'power') by implying that the NP, in this respect, does not have a greater level or access to knowledge than the patient.

Other ways that advice is mitigated throughout this exchange come in a number of lexical and syntactic choices. For example, the use of the term "surveillance" (lines 23, 25 and 33) rather than "annual check-up" or "annual testing with a urologist," which would be more specific, has a similar effect as "every now and then" in minimizing the sense of imposition on the patient. Laura's advice also includes passive voice in line 43: "a PSA needs to be done" in which Mr. Vaughn's role in this action is silenced, thereby minimizing his role and any imposition on him that this might involve. Similarly, in lines 61 and 63, Laura frames the advice with "I think," which Leech refers to as strategy for "hedging advice" (2014, p. 207). Later in the excerpt, Laura uses "kinda" (line 67) and "just" (lines 67, 68, 73 and 83) to minimize the force of the advice which she this time refers to as "touch(ing) base," suggesting a brief rather than long, in-depth meeting. Finally, in line 90, where the advice is most direct, it is presented as a desire in her choice of "you want" rather than an obligation such as "you should." Any one of these mitigating devices has the effect of lessening the intensity of the imposition; however, taken together over the course of a number of turns, the effect is much greater.

Another feature of this advice-giving sequence is the explanation Laura gives for her medical advice. Unlike the urologist that Mr. Vaughn alludes to who did not provide a clear justification for why he should continue to see him (referenced in lines 36–40), Laura provides justification, sometimes fairly vague as in the case of "surveillance," sometimes more specific, for example, her explanation in lines 74–77. Justification for the advice is given in lines 22–23, 67–70 and 74–77. Providing a rationale for this medical advice is reminiscent of Peräkylä's (1998) evidential diagnostic claims in that it seems to add both authority and accountability to Laura's advice to resume the urology visits. It is also a way of educating the patient, similar to the kind of knowledge sharing discussed in Chap. 3.

3.4 A Short Spike Every Now and Then Is Okay

In the prior excerpt, it is clear through the uptake that the patient was able to accurately interpret the advice; moreover, it is not surprising since the advice was on record. Therefore, the use of indirectness did not necessarily jeopardize the message being communicated accurately. However, in the following excerpt, the NP, Julie, takes a greater risk of the implicature not going through by using off-record indirectness to advise the patient, Mr. Adams, to not continue taking a particular medication. She does this in the form of educating him (lines 6–15) about how he should interpret his blood pressure and what the appropriate response is (or in this case, is not). Within this explanation, there is not only the off-record advice, but also an implicit critique of his past behavior of going against another provider's advice.

Mr. Adams is a first-time patient for Julie and is at the visit to check medications following cardiac surgery a few months prior. Julie spends most of the visit identifying Mr. Adams' medications and adjusting and refilling medications as needed. Early in the visit, Mr. Adams explains that he was told by another provider to stop taking his blood pressure medicine, but after only a couple of days, he started taking it again because his "blood pressure ran up" and he "started feelin' funny in the head." Julie responds to this by using off-record indirectness with no reference to either the medication or the advice (e.g. don't take the blood pressure medicine because you don't actually need it). Instead, she leaves it up to Mr. Adams to get the intended meaning of her utterance, possibly relying on his familiarity with the context and the prior discourse to get the intended meaning.

Excerpt 4

1. Julie: um hang on I'm gonna give you back the ni- nifedipine
2.   this is the one you to you resumed this is that brown
3.   [one right?
4. Mr. Adams: [that brown one right there started takin' it [again
5. Julie: [ye:ah um so
6.   just to let you know blood pressure going up to one
7.   thirty-eight or even one forty that's okay (.) I mean
8.   when I looked in your book overall there was only a
9.   few times it went up that high and sometimes if we're um
10.   not feeling well or if we're stressed or um anxious
11.   about anything our blood pressure might naturally
12.   rise a little bit and that's okay if your blood pressure
13.   was consistently staying higher, then we'd want to
14.   make sure we gave you something for it but (.) a
15.   short spike every now and then is okay (1.0) um let's see...

Similar to the previous example, Julie starts with a question in line 2: "you resumed... that brown one right," which requests clarification identifying the medication Mr. Adams resumed. Since it has already been determined that Mr. Adams resumed taking this medication that another provider told him to stop taking, we cannot interpret this question as 'pre-advice' since presumably Julie would give the advice independent of Mr. Adams' response to the question. She might delay the advice until she identified which colored pill the blood pressure medication is, but as noted, the fact that he resumed the blood pressure medication is, at this point, given information. The advice, then starts at line 6 and comprises the rest of Julie's turn (lines 6–15). It begins with an elongated "yeah," acting as a turn initiator and "pivot" from listener to speaker role (Drummond & Hopper, 1993, p. 205), includes a turn initial "so," indicating a shift from the previous topic (Schiffrin, 1988), and a hesitation marker "um," marking the discourse as either difficult for the speaker or important for the listener (Fox Tree & Clark, 2002). Julie then begins the advice with "just to let you know," which has the locutionary effect of prefacing information sharing, a part of advice-giving. She also includes specific blood pressure readings: 138 and 140, which are the readings Mr. Adams previously claimed were too high, causing him to restart the medication. In line 9, as part of the advice-giving, Julie uses the all-inclusive "we," meaning something akin to 'all humans' to explain how blood pressure may fluctuate and why the numbers he mentioned are not necessarily problematic or cause for concern. The combination of using the numbers he provided earlier with the more general use of "we" hints at the advice without explicitly stating it. Julie is relying on Mr. Adams to draw the connection between the numbers he mentioned and the more general patterns Julie describes to recognize that he should not worry about a blood pressure reading of 138 or 140 and that it is not a cause for concern or a reason to go against a provider's advice. In line 14, she comes close to referencing his medication but uses the nonspecific term "something"; however, this is still off record since there is no deictic (i.e. this/that medication) or reference to the medication he stopped. An utterance such as "we'd put you back on that," for instance, could be considered on record since reference to the particular medication can be inferred.

In this excerpt, there is no clear uptake from the patient. There is a one-second pause before Julie moves on to the next topic, so it is possible that Mr. Adams provides a nonverbal response or acknowledgement of the advice; however, without visual data, it is impossible to confirm this. Overall, Julie does not provide a significant amount of time to allow Mr. Adams to respond nor does she prompt a response from him in any way, something like 'okay?' or 'does that make sense?' both of which may be too direct, particularly in combination with the off-record form that the advice takes in this example. It is possible that Julie is relying on the context of the medical setting, her role as medical provider and his role as patient, to disambiguate her turn and recognize it as advice to follow the instructions of his providers.

In this example, Julie also avoids directly criticizing Mr. Adams' decision to go against his physician's advice to stop taking his blood pressure medication by presenting it as a general statement about what one should not do rather than admonishing him for ignoring his provider's directions and making the decision on his own to resume taking the medication. It is not clear from the discourse whether one of the reasons for this is because of possible adverse effects it was having, for example, lowering his potassium levels, something that Julie discusses as a concern with other patients; therefore, the stakes of Mr. Adams' decision to take the referenced medication are not entirely clear. As mentioned, off-record indirectness involves the greatest risk of the intended message not going through; therefore, it is surprising that NPs would use this tactic. The additional speech act of critiquing past behavior may account for the off-record form that this advice/critique takes.

3.5 A Lot of People Do It This Way

The final example of indirectness actually involves multiple tactics that have been discussed so far as well as the use of voicing non-present others as a way of providing advice. In the example presented below, June takes on the voice of a set of hypothetical patients. In this case, it is unlikely that "a lot of people" (line 6) actually uttered the same thing; instead, June seems to be taking on the identity of these other patients as a model with which Ms. Lambert, the patient, is invited to either align or disalign. This excerpt has been discussed in detail elsewhere (Defibaugh, 2014), where I show that the pattern of June voicing others is a productive form of indirect advice for her. Here, I will focus on the ways that it performs the function of both critique and advice while distancing both June and Ms. Lambert through the hypothetical speech of non-present others.

Excerpt 5

1. June: you would never wanna run out of the blood pressure
2. medicine,
3. Ms. Lambert: no
4. June: you would never wanna run out of the diabetes medicine
5. Ms. Lambert: sure don't and be back [in this situation
6. June: [and A LOT OF PEOPLE do
7. it this way they say we:ll (.) I've got medicine for three
8. different things, what's the big deal if I take medicine
9. for two out of the three things and it's a really big deal
10. Ms. Lambert: mmhmm
11. June: 'cuz what you've got is thi- I want you to think of it
12. this way you've got all these dinner plates and they
13. all have to be held up you can't drop the diabetes
14. one (1.0) and think that its gonna be okay: and
15. you can't drop the (.) blood pressure one and think
16. that everything's gonna be okay you can't drop
17. the cholesterol one (.) so you're holding up all
18. these dinner plates and they're all of equal importance
19. Ms. Lambert: okay

The excerpt begins with June giving on-record advice with the use of a hedged, hypothetical phrase, "you would never wanna" (lines 1 and 4). This is similar to the tactic employed by Laura who also uses hedging to give advice (excerpt 3). This hypothetical future advice could be given to someone such as Mr. Bray, who has just been diagnosed with diabetes. It isn't until Ms. Lambert's uptake in line 5 that it is clear that she is not newly diagnosed but instead is in the hospital due to poor management of her disease. When Ms. Lambert says, "sure don't and be back in this situation," she acknowledges that this is not only future advice but also a critique of her past behavior, which she readily admits. The critique then comes, first, in June's on-record indirect advice about not wanting to run out of any of her medications. The advice/critique then continues when June voices other patients in lines 7–9. She voices the bad patient who does not take all three of his/her medications and sees this is as not a "big deal" (line 8). She then counters these hypothetical patients by returning to her own voice and stating, "it's a really big deal" (line 9). The advice comes in the form of creating a possible juxtaposition for Ms. Lambert between what she "wants to do" in the future compared to what "a lot of people do." Based on the context, Ms. Lambert is like "a lot of people" in that she has failed to see all three of her medications as of "equal importance" (line 18), which is why June starts by referencing both the blood pressure and the diabetes medicine (lines 1–2 and 4), refers to the hypothetical patients as taking "three things" (line 9), and then, within the metaphor of someone holding up three dinner plates, again makes explicit what those three things are "the diabetes one" (lines 13–14), "the blood pressure one" (line 15), and "the cholesterol one" (line 17).

Similar to June's use of directness with Mr. Bray (excerpt 1), she uses the imperative "you can't drop" in reference to the hypothetical dinner plates (lines 11–18). In the earlier example, the imperative was in reference to vague advice of "concentrate your efforts" where the more explicit advice came later in a different clause, separate from the imperative. Here, she uses the imperative with respect to the medications but within the loosely veiled metaphor of holding up dinner plates. The patient then must make the connections between the hypothetical future actions of "you don't want to," the non-present, hypothetical bad patients and the metaphorical person holding up three dinner plates, which all must be balanced to recognize the critique of past behavior as well as the advice for future actions. Here, unlike in excerpt 4, the intended meaning seems much more obvious, both because of its on-record nature in mentioning of the medications and in the repetition of advice through various, albeit, indirect means.

4 Conclusion

In this chapter, I have outlined a number of ways in which NPs use indirect speech to give medical directives and advice, and in some cases, to critique patients' past behavior as well. Together, these examples illustrate a range in which indirectness may be employed when giving medical advice to patients. One tactic, for example, is June's use of the direct imperative only with general, nonspecific advice. In the case of Mr. Bray, she gives a vague imperative but follows it up with the specific advice in a separate clause. With Ms. Lambert, June uses the imperative within the frame of the dinner plate metaphor. The specific kinds of medication are not mentioned within the imperative clause; instead, she refers to them using the indefinite "one" (i.e. the diabetes one) where "one" references the dinner plates directly but also, by extension, makes reference to medications. Karen, similarly, uses a direct imperative when telling Mr. Eggers where to purchase the vitamin supplement, but in doing so she is also giving the advice that he needs to take the medicine. This is mostly clearly seen in the way that she follows up the second imperative, "make sure you buy that" with an explanation that is about his need for the medication rather than the financial benefit of buying it over the counter rather than with a prescription.

The more indirect forms seem to occur more frequently when the utterance also has the additional, bivalent meaning of criticism for poor health choices in the past, which is not surprising since a criticism involves a threat to the patient's positive face in addition to the threat to a patient's negative face that directives entail. Laura uses extensive mitigation, hedging, and justification in response to Mr. Vaughn's claim that he has not seen a urologist in years (excerpt 3) to both indirectly criticize his lapse in visiting the urologist as well as advise him to make an appointment and resume these annual visits. Julie uses off-record indirectness, again to criticize and advise Mr. Adams about his resuming his blood pressure medication when another provider told him to stop taking it. This is the least transparent of the advice included in this chapter and the only one that lacks clear acknowledgement by the patient that the intended message went through. The final example includes multiple indirectness tactics: the use of a hypothetical future event of running out of medication (through the use of the modal 'would'), voicing a set of 'bad' patients who do not understand the importance of taking all of their medications, and employment of the dinner plate metaphor, discussed above.

The reasons that these NPs use indirectness when giving medical advice may be attributed to their enactment of their professional competency and their focus on patient-centered care. By minimizing the force of the directive through various indirect means, NPs lessen the possible face threats to patients, making the medical advice seem more like suggestions rather than directives, thereby giving patients a greater sense of autonomy. This diminishing of FTA is one way in which NPs can perform relational work, attending to the management of provider–patient relationships, and, as most of the examples indicate, without concern of being misinterpreted. As mentioned, the only example in which there is no clear patient uptake of the message is when off-record indirectness is used. In this case, it may be more important for Julie to maintain a positive relationship with the patient rather than insisting upon a particular course of action. In each of the instances, indirectness seems to support a positive provider–patient relationship through lowering the sense of hierarchical power and lowering the sense of imposition on the patient.

Notes

1. 'Can you X?' and similar question-formulated directives are so conventionalized for speakers of American English that many do not necessarily view this as an indirect form. It does, however, meet the criteria for Searle in that the literal meaning is a question of the hearer's ability while the implicated meaning is a request for the hearer to perform the action.

References

American Society for Clinical Oncology. (2017). *Follow up for prostate cancer.* Retrieved July 28, 2017, from http://www.cancer.net/research-and-advocacy/asco-care-and-treatment-recommendations-patients/follow-care-prostate-cancer

Benkendorf, J. L., Prince, M. B., Rose, M. A., De Fina, A., & Hamilton, H. E. (2001). Does indirect speech promote nondirective genetic counseling? Results of a sociolinguistic investigation. *American Journal of Medical Genetics, 106,* 199–207.

Bonnefon, J. F., Feeney, A., & De Neys, W. (2011). The risk of polite misunderstandings. *Current Directions in Psychological Science, 20*(5), 321–324.

Brown, P., & Levinson, S. (1987). *Universals in language usage: Politeness phenomena.* Cambridge: Cambridge University Press.

Caffi, C. (1999). On mitigation. *Journal of Pragmatics, 31,* 881–909.

Defibaugh, S. (2014). Management of health or management of face: Indirectness in nurse practitioner-patient interactions. *Journal of Pragmatics, 67,* 61–71.
Drummond, K., & Hopper, R. (1993). Some uses of yeah. *Research on Language and Social Interaction, 26*(2), 203–212.
Fox Tree, J. E., & Clark, H. H. (2002). Using 'uh' and 'um' in spontaneous speaking. *Cognition, 84,* 73–111.
Goffman, E. (1967). *Interaction ritual: Essays of face-to-face behavior.* Garolen City, NY: Anchor/Doubleday.
Haugh, M. (2015). *Im/politeness and implicatures.* New York: Mouton de Gruyter.
Kiesling, S. F., & Johnson, E. G. (2010). Four forms of interactional indirection. *Journal of Pragmatics, 42,* 292–306.
Leech, G. (2014). *Pragmatics of politeness.* Oxford: Oxford University Press.
Lempert, M. (2012). Indirectness. In C. Paulston, S. Kiesling, & E. Rangel (Eds.), *The handbook of intercultural discourse and communication.* Wiley Blackwell.
Levinson, S. (1983). *Pragmatics.* Cambridge: Cambridge University Press.
Morgan, M. H. (1991). Indirectness and interpretation in African American women's discourse. *Pragmatics, 1*(4), 421–451.
Parry, R. (2005). A video analysis of how physiotherapists communicate with patients about errors of performance: Insights for practice and policy. *Physiotherapy, 91,* 204–214.
Peräkylä, A. (1998). Authority and accountability: The delivery of diagnosis in primary health care. *Social Psychology Quarterly, 61*(4), 301–320.
Schiffrin, D. (1988). *Discourse markers.* Cambridge: Cambridge University Press.
Schneider. (2010). Mitigaion. In M. A. Locher & S. L. Graham (Eds.), *Interpersonal pragmatics* (pp. 253–270). Berlin: De Gruyter Mouton.
Searle, J. (1975). Indirect speech acts. In P. Cole & J. Morgan (Eds.), *Syntax and semantics* (pp. 59–82).
Tannen, D. (2010). Abduction and identity in family interaction: Ventriloquizing as indirectness. *Journal of Pragmatics, 42,* 307–316.
Thaler, V. (2012). Mitigation as modification of illocutionary force. *Journal of Pragmatics, 44,* 907–919.
Thomas, J. (1986). *The dynamics of discourse: A pragmatic analysis of confrontational interaction,* Unpublished Doctoral Dissertation. University of Lancaster, Lancaster, UK.

CHAPTER 5

Caring as Competent: Small Talk in Medical Visits

Abstract Small talk in medical visits affords the opportunity for nurse practitioners (NPs) and patients to create relationships by engaging in nontransactional talk. In addition, it may also provide insights into a patient's life, revealing medically relevant information. Although small talk may be viewed as taking time away from the transactional work of the visit (Roter & Hall, Doctors talking with patients/patients talking with doctors: Improving communication in medical visits, Praeger, 1993), it is also a way for NPs to perform their professional competency by taking a holistic approach and constructing positive relationships. Small talk, despite being a departure from the transactional work of the visit, can also contribute to it.

Keywords Frames • Transactional/interactional • Goal-oriented/ socially oriented talk • Personal engagement • Provider–patient relationships

1 INTRODUCTION

This chapter outlines the ways in which nurse practitioners (NPs) perform their professional competency through engagement in small talk (e.g. relational talk). Small talk, although primarily a departure from the medical goals of the visit, can be understood as accomplishing interactional goals as it allows NPs to create positive provider–patient relationships and treat patients from a personal, holistic perspective. Although small talk may be viewed as taking time away from the transactional work of the visit, such as engaging in patient education or allowing time for discussion of treatment options (Roter & Hall, 1992), I illustrate how small talk does not necessarily require a great deal of time but may be worthwhile in contributing to overall positive health outcomes. I draw on prior research on small talk in institutional and workplace settings as well as in medical visits and argue that small talk that occurs at various points in the visit does contribute to the overall transactional work rather than taking away from it. This chapter presents four extracts from different medical visits in which the provider and patient, or in the case of the last example, the patient's wife, engage in small talk. The first two are from an initial exchange, at the beginning of the visit, which, I argue creates rapport that may extend through the rest of the visit. The second occurs during a transitional point in the visit and illustrates how small talk may include medically relevant information while still attending to interpersonal goals. The final example of small talk is from a closing sequence, in which the transactional goals of the visit are complete. In this case, small talk may allow for the creation of positive relationships that extend beyond the individual visit and set up an ongoing relationship for future care.

2 Defining Small Talk

Small talk has been a focus of linguistic inquiry for decades. Often aligned to Malinowski's "phatic communion," which he defines as "a type of speech in which ties of union are created by a mere exchange of words" (1923, reproduced in N. Coupland & Jaworski, 2006, p. 297), small talk, by nature, has the primary function of a social rather than informational exchange. Malinowski includes such topics as "inquiries about health, comments on weather" and "affirmations of some supremely obvious state of things" (296) in his description of phatic communion, illustrating its purely relational focus.

Since Malinowski, others have attempted various definitions of small talk. Maynard and Hudak (2008), with a focus on institutional settings, consider goal orientation in the distinction between small talk and 'work talk.' They argue that small talk is interpersonal, relational, and lacking in goal orientation; work talk, on the other hand, is transactional, instrumental, and goal-oriented. This distinction between interactional and transactional is one which is useful in analyzing talk in institutional settings such as medical visits in which talk is often goal-oriented; interactional talk can then be understood as departures from the goal-oriented, transactional talk. Despite the apparently clear delineation that the terminology suggests, as others have noted, it is not so easy make this distinction. Koester argues, "even talk at work which seems to bear no relation to any task at hand may have some relevance, even indirect to other workplace interactions" (2010, p. 15), for example, in creating group cohesion, lowering the social barriers between supervisor and subordinates, or contributing to the development of workplace relationships, particularly in supplier–customer interactions (see Koester, 2010, Chap. 5 for more on this topic). Coupland (2000), similarly, points out how small talk cannot be neatly separated from other types of talk, particularly in workplace and institutional settings because these types of talk can bleed into one another. For example, Coupland claims that in medical encounters, "talk about social circumstances and family connections may trigger discussion of environmental matters which could be relevant to the clinic's and the doctor's professional responsibilities" (2000, p. 22). That is, small talk may reveal important details that are relevant to the work at hand. In this way, small talk, although not goal-*oriented*, could be transactional in some respects and contribute to institutional goals.

Holmes (2000), likewise, argues against a clear and simple delineation between small talk and work talk. Rather than seeing these as possibly overlapping in their goal orientation, she views these as two ends of a continuum of talk, where any particular exchange may fall somewhere along it. On the far left of the continuum, she places "core business talk"; on the far right, "phatic communion,'" with the more marginal categories of "social talk" and "work-related talk" falling in between these two. Viewing talk as existing along a continuum means that talk can fall into a particular category, such as 'social talk' or 'core business talk' or could lie somewhere in between, having certain characteristics of each. This perspective also suggests that the categories of work talk and small talk are too simplistic and ignore the fact that talk can, to varying extents, address both transactional and interactional goals. Holmes also distinguishes "social talk" from "phatic communion," suggesting that small does not just include Malinowski's list of seemingly insignificant topics but instead represents a broader category of relationally focused talk. In the same vein, Koester (2010) also considers phatic communion to be its own category within the larger set of what she terms "relational talk." In her analysis of workplace discourse, she views relational talk as being more than simply phatic communion, which she defines as being talk that happens only at the "edges" of encounters and are based on ritual exchanges (Laver, 1975, cited in Koester, 2010). Koester includes the following three categories, in addition to phatic communion, as types of relational talk: (1) "non-transactional conversations," which can be understood as quintessential small talk that occurs elsewhere, beyond the 'edges'; (2) "relational episodes" in which small talk overlaps with transactional tasks; and (3) "relational sequences and turns" or "non-obligatory task-related talk with a relational focus" (97). Koester's categories make important distinctions in terms of where small talk occurs within an exchange, the extent to which it may overlap or be integrated into the work of transactional tasks, and the way that it may occur in relative isolation from work-related tasks and talk. Although relational talk is just one aspect of her examination of workplace discourse, she argues that workers engage in a great deal of relational talk and that it is just as important as transactional talk in terms of both participation in workplace settings and our study of them.

Despite the general frequency of small talk in institutional or workplace settings, Koester (2010) notes that the actual workplace setting may influence the degree to which small talk is found. She notes that different types of service encounters often involve more or less relational talk. For example, more service-oriented settings such as interactions in hair salons or exchanges between driving instructors and students (McCarthy, 2000) often involve more small talk compared to more task-oriented interactions, such as responding to emergency calls (Zimmerman, 1992), the difference being the extent to which relational talk may overlap with other work-related tasks. Driving instructions, for example, may be given when necessary, and when there is silence, it may be filled with small talk. In the case of emergency calls, there is no 'down time' in which participants are not actively attending to the goal orientation of the call. Nonemergency medical visits, such as the ones in the book, fall somewhere in the middle in terms of the degree to which the talk is task oriented compared to relationally oriented and the extent to which relational talk may overlap with transactional tasks. The following section outlines a number of key studies in the analysis of small talk in medical visits.

2.1 Small Talk in Medical Visits

A number of researchers have discussed the role of small talk in medical encounters (Coupland, 2000; Coupland, Robinson, & Coupland, 1994; Defibaugh, in press; Hudak & Maynard, 2011; Maynard & Hudak, 2008; Ragan, 2000) including considerations of the form that small talk takes (Hudak & Maynard, 2011) and the functions that it has within medical visits (Coupland et al., 1994; Defibaugh, in press; Maynard & Hudak, 2008; Ragan, 2000). In this section, I highlight three of these studies which are particularly relevant to the discussion of small talk as a function of professional competency. These three studies represent the range in which researchers may consider small talk as having a transactional function in addition to the relational one. Maynard and Hudak (2008) discuss small talk as functioning outside the transactional work of the visit. Coupland et al. (1994) consider the potential duality that small talk can perform, while Ragan (2000) illustrates how a particular kind of small talk can directly aid in the transactional goals of the visit.

As noted in the previous section, Maynard and Hudak (2008) primarily view small talk as a departure from work talk; that is, small talk is not goal oriented and is separate in its function from the more goal-oriented, transactional talk that occurs in medical visits. They argue that both providers and patients may use small talk to 'disattend' to the medical visit. They make a distinction between "disattending," which they define as an effort "to push instrumental tasks of various kinds to the background" (662) of the medical visit, and "inattentiveness," which suggests a lack of concern or attention by one or both of the parties to the transactional goals of the visit. They identify two ways in which small talk can 'disattend' to the instrumental tasks. The first is "disattentiveness-in-simultaneity," or instances of small talk that co-occur but not necessarily align with instrumental tasks, including small talk that occurs while a provider is looking through a patient's chart at the beginning of the visit, or during transitional phases of the visit when both participants are not just interactionally but also physically realigning to the next phase or task, for example, moving from the desk to the examination table or back. The second type they describe is "disattentiveness-in-sequence," or the ways in which both patient and provider may use small talk as a tool to shift the talk away from the instrumental task, described particularly as a topic-avoidance strategy. One example they give of this is a doctor responding to a patient's negative assessment of the cost of a prescribed medication. Rather than responding to this complaint, which is phased as a negative polarity question ("I don't suppose the insurance will cover that," p. 679), the provider lightheartedly suggests that the patient contact a state representative and/or the US president to get that changed. This light-hearted shift works, they note, as the patient then shifts topics to talk about how she knows one of the representative's relatives. What this study highlights is that although small talk is separate from work talk, it can perform no transactional functions within the visit, making it important in its own right.

Another significant contribution to the research on small talk in medical visits is Coupland, Robinson, and Coupland's (1994) examination of small talk during openings of geriatric medical visits in the United Kingdom. They focus specifically on what they term HAY? or the various forms of *how are you* questions that occur during the opening phase of the medical visit. Unlike Maynard and Hudak (2008), who view small talk as separate from the transactional work of the visit, Coupland and colleagues argue that "even wholly relationally focused exchanges" are important sites of transactional work (1994, p. 94). For example, they note that a patient's willingness to engage in small talk may indicate their general attitude, health or morale, which the provider can then use as a guide to the rest of the visit. Additionally, information that arises in small talk exchanges can give important health insights into the patient's family life and social support or provide topics that the provider may want to draw on later in the visit. They give the example of a provider complimenting a patient's gold bracelet, which indirectly brings up other topics, such as the patient's children and alcohol, both of which may be medically relevant. Finally, they also note that small talk such as compliments, teasing, familiarity sequences, and other phatic communion lays the groundwork for a relationship that involves "*genuine*, personal involvement and concern" (102), which allows for a lowered sense of face threats when it comes to the more medically focused talk that occurs later in the visit. Therefore, by showing apparent "genuine" interest in the patient, the provider can frame medical advice more effectively as being in the patient's best interest, which the provider has shown to be concerned about through engaging in relationally focused exchanges. Coupland et al. (1994) use the concept of "frames," or what Tannen refers to as "structures of expectation" (1993, p. 21) to explain shifts between small talk and work talk. Small talk exchanges are described as being primarily within a "socio-relational frame," or a set of expectations for interpersonal exchanges, rather than a "medical frame," which would draw participants into more medically relevant interactional exchanges. The authors claim that even though these are two different frames, the socio-relational frame can allow for negotiation into the medical frame, making it integral to the transactional work of the visit in a multitude of ways.

Ragan's (2000) study of small talk in medical visits goes even one step further by making explicit the role that small talk can play in the transactional work of the visit. She provides an example in which a female provider, during gynecology visits, shares personal stories of her own medical care including personal use of medications as a way to provide advice for the patient. In this way, she argues that "sociable talk" is not a departure from work talk but an essential aspect of it:

> Sociable talk, i.e. relational communication between provider and patient is tantamount to the task, in that the 'task' of these health-care interactions is not merely to interview, examine, diagnose and treat/proscribe; it is also to co-create a relational climate that facilitates these critical medical achievements. (269)

Ragan's example is an interesting one as it more clearly crosses the boundary between work talk and small talk, falling somewhere between "social talk" and "work-related talk" (Holmes, 2000). It is also in line with Koester's (2010) "relational sequences and turns," in which the social talk contributes to the work talk rather directly.

As these studies illustrate, small talk is an integral part of medical care. Although primarily understood as relational work, small talk can do additional transaction work as well. Defibaugh (in press) argues that because small talk can be understood as primarily relational and allows for rapport-building between provider and patient, even seemingly purely relational talk can enhance the provider–patient relationship, making it an important component of patient-centered health care. On the other hand, Roter and Hall (1992) caution that "too much social conversation may take visit time away from information giving and counseling on the part of the physician and make it more difficult for the patient to provide the important psychosocial and biomedical information that provides insight into his or her illness experience and medication condition" (91). In the data presented in the following section, three of the four examples of small talk are relatively short and do not take any substantial amount of time away from the more transactionally focused aspects of the visits. The third example is rather lengthy but occurs at the end of the visit, when the transactional work is completed (see Defibaugh, in press for a similar example and a more comprehensive discussion of extended small talk in closings).

3 SMALL TALK ACROSS THE SPAN OF THE VISIT

Following Coupland et al. (1994), I employ the concept of frames, noting two frames of interaction: the relational frame and the medical frame, although, as I illustrate, these are not necessarily competing frames. That is, the relational frame may still contribute to the medical tasks. Instead, it is a matter of orientation of the talk, with the difference being whether participants appear to be orienting their talk and responses to each other within a relational/social frame or a medical frame. Talk within the relational frame typically involves participants orienting to their noninstitutional identities of provider or patient and drawing on aspects of their identities outside of the medical encounter. The medical frame is noted by talk that is medically focused and related to the goals of the visit. By interacting within both the relational and the medical frame, NPs and patients are able create a provider–patient relationship while still attending to the medical tasks of the visit.

The following data excerpts come from four outpatient visits in the Veterans Affairs (VA) clinic and involve all three NPs (Laura, Karen, and Sarah) working at that location. All the visits took place during the week before and the week of Thanksgiving. Because of this, there is a reference to the 'holidays,' a discussion about Thanksgiving preparation, and a gift from a patient of Serbian nut bread, likely a result of the holiday season, when individuals in the United States are more likely to give gifts of homemade sweets and pastries. Because all of the excerpts in this chapter occur just before the Thanksgiving holiday, it could be argued that these are atypical and that small talk is influenced by the holiday itself. However, I would argue that while the topic of the small talk in each visit may be influenced by the holiday, the existence of small talk is not limited to just this topic and likely not just this time of year. As many other researchers have noted, small talk occurs somewhat frequently in medical visits; furthermore, as excerpt 3 illustrates, not all small talk is centered around the topic of Thanksgiving. In Defibaugh (in press), I provide an additional example of extended small talk that occurs at the end of the visit in which the topic is not based around the holidays but on family pets.

The small talk examples in this chapter are presented based on where they occur in the visit and illustrate a range of functions that the small talk performs. The first two illustrate how small talk at the beginning of the visit creates rapport for both the NP and the patient. In the first of these two, Laura engages in minimal small talk with the patient while setting up for his visit; in the second, the patient seemingly creates rapport with his NP, Karen, through the use of humor and discussion of a gift he brought her. In both excerpts, the small talk is relatively brief before the NP then shifts frames by focusing on the transactional aspects of the visit. The third example, also involving Karen, illustrates small talk that occurs in the middle of the visit. It is a very brief departure from the work of the visit as most of the discussion can be understood as medically relevant. The departure, however, shows an interest in the patient beyond simply his general health. The fourth and final example of small talk is much longer than the others. It occurs at the end of the visit and demonstrates how the NP, Sarah, continues to create rapport with the patient and his spouse even after the medical goals of the visit have been accomplished. Each of these examples represent slightly different uses of small talk; however, each can be understood as an effort at rapport-building and as an enactment of the patient-centered approach.

3.1 Are You All Ready for the Holidays?

The first example of small talk is quite brief but illustrates how the NP begins the medical visit by attempting to create rapport with the patient. This excerpt is taken from an outpatient visit in the VA clinic between Laura and Mr. Vaughn. Mr. Vaughn is a long-term patient for Laura but one that she sees only for the annual visit. Laura's questions in lines 1 and 5 both illustrate efforts at relational talk that is prior to and separate from the transactional focus of the visit.

Excerpt 1

1. Laura: how are you:
2. Mr. Vaughn: fine thank you
3. Laura: good good
4. Mr. Vaughn: yeah (1.0)
5. Laura: all right so are you all ready for the holidays?
6. Mr. Vaughn: all ready

7. Laura: good let me just take care of this other gentleman
8. ordering meds and then I'll be right with you
9. Mr. Vaughn: okay fine fine
10. Laura: and then we'll go over all of your bloodwork and you'll
11. get a copy of it
12. Mr. Vaughn: okay

In this excerpt, Laura begins with a HAY? (e.g. *how are you?* Coupland et al., 1994), which could be interpreted as either a general, phatic question or a legitimate question of one's health due to the institutional setting, the former indicating a relational frame, and the latter, a medical frame. In this case, the stress and elongated final vowel on "you" (line 1) seems to indicate a relational frame, which cues the patient to this being an attempt at phatic communion rather than a question about his overall health. The patient's response of "fine thank you" (line 2) suggests that this was his interpretation as well. Laura then, rather than moving from relational to transactional talk, asks another social question: "so are you all ready for the holidays?" (line 5). Unlike the HAY?, this question is unambiguous in its focus on relational talk and provides the patient with an opportunity to share information about his life. Rather than taking this opportunity, he provides only a brief response (line 6), likely orienting to the medical question and answer sequence of turn-taking, as discussed in Chap. 2, suggesting a lack of desire to engage in the relational frame. Laura's use of small talk questions at the beginning of this visit performs a number of functions. First, as Coupland et al. (1994) note, small talk allows a provider to create a friendly rapport and atmosphere for the patient by engaging in non-work talk at the outset. There is also an opportunity for a patient to share more of what is happening in his/her personal life (although, in this case, the patient does not take this opportunity) which the provider can draw on later in the visit. Finally, as is evidenced from her turn in line 7, Laura is using small talk in order to multitask. As NPs in this clinic see patients in back-to-back 30-minute intervals, she did not have time to complete the tasks from the previous visit prior to Mr. Vaughn's arrival in her office. By asking him about his holidays, there is potential to fill this silence while she completes the electronic prescriptions for the previous patient. Laura's use of small talk performs a kind of "disattentiveness-in-simultaneity" (Maynard & Hudak, 2008), but in this case, it is transitioning between visits rather than between phases in an individual visit.

3.2 They Said I Go Next to See the Boss

The second excerpt also occurs at the beginning of the visit. Similar to the exchange between Laura and Mr. Vaughn, Karen begins the visit with a HAY? that the patient responds to minimally. However, the patient, Mr. Griffin, upgrades the relational talk by using humor (lines 4 & 6) and by offering Karen a gift of Serbian nut bread, which is the focus of talk in lines 9–16. Following this exchange, Mr. Griffin shifts the talk to the transactional focus of the visit in line 19 by offering Karen his medical paperwork to review, moving from a relational to a medical frame.

Excerpt 2

1. Karen: hi Mr. Griffin how are: you:
2. Mr. Griffin: I'm okay
3. Karen: have a seat [nice to see you
4. Mr. Griffin: okay   [they said I they said I go next to see the boss
5. Karen: hhhhhh they call me the boss?
6. Mr. Griffin: that's what they said
7. Karen: that's pretty sweet of them haven't seen you in a year but
8. you certainly lookin' good
9. Mr. Griffin: ah: let's see I don't know if you want any of these that's
10. frozen that povitica I don't know if you've ever heard of that
11. Karen: what is it?
12. Mr. Griffin: povitica its ### and Serbian for ah nut bread
13. Karen: oh: pumpkin
14. Mr. Griffin: yeah
15. Karen: oh my god my family loves pumpkin bread thank you so
16. much you didn't have to do that
17. Mr. Griffin: could you hang this somewhere
18. Karen: yes I will hang it up for you no problem
19. Mr. Griffin: well anyway here's some old stuff I don't if-
20. Karen: have you been in the hospital at all in the past year

Karen begins the exchange with a typical HAY? As indicated in the transcript, this is produced with elongated vowels on both "are" and "you," suggesting a relational frame and a genuineness in her concern and interest in Mr. Griffin, whose response of "okay" (line 2) reflects a phatic interpretation rather than a medical inquiry. Karen continues the relational talk with her utterance of "nice to see you" (line 3), which references a familiarity with the patient and a prior relationship. As she notes, she has not seen Mr. Griffin since the previous year as he is also a patient who only comes in for his annual checkup. The patient then upgrades this relational exchange by using humor, referring to her as "the boss" (line 4). He does this through constructed dialogue of, presumably, Karen's nurse who brings the patients to her after the initial check-in. The reference to "the boss" is clearly intended to be humorous but acknowledges both the power asymmetry between them as well as a kind of familiarity. Mr. Griffin simultaneously references Karen's higher position of institutional power in the exchange but also creates rapport with her by making this joke, both of which suggest a measure of familiarity between the two. Karen laughs and continues this line of joking with him before shifting to a statement, "you certainly lookin' good" (line 8) that seems to skirt the line between relational and transactional, as it could be understood as a reference to his health. However, the conversational, informal way this is stated, in which the verb is omitted (as compared to the more formal 'you *are* looking good'), suggests a continuation of the relational frame by Karen. Although Mr. Griffin does not respond to this comment, he continues in the relational frame by offering her a gift of Serbian nut bread ("povitica"), which is the focus of discussion in lines 9–16. Karen later commented to me how nice it was that he brought this to her, suggesting that this is not typical in this clinic and likely due to the timing of the visit just days before Thanksgiving. There is then some discussion of where Mr. Griffin can hang his coat (17–18), which is then followed by Mr. Griffin's move at transitioning to the transactional focus of the visit. In line 19, he references his paperwork from medical care received over the past year: "well anyway here's some old stuff" (19), offering them to Karen to review and add to his medical records with the VA. His use of "well anyway" at the beginning of this turn signals a reorientation in the discourse (Fraser, 1988); in this case, it is an orientation to the medical frame that the patient likely expects by this point in the visit and of which he likely recognizes his role in the departure from in the prior discourse. Karen then solidifies the move into the medical frame with her question about Mr. Griffin's possible hospitalization (line 20).

These two excerpts illustrate how both the NP and the patient may orient and contribute to the relational frame at the beginning of the visit. In the case of excerpt 1, Laura offers two relationally focused questions, which Mr. Vaughn responds to minimally. Her use of small talk here is an example of "disattentiveness-in-simultaneity" (Maynard & Hudak, 2008), offering the patient an opportunity to share information about himself while she is finishing up work from the prior visit. The second example begins quite similarly, but in this case, the patient upgrades the relational talk by making a joke and offering the NP a gift. For both, small talk is relatively short and takes very little time away from the visit, which seems to be within the "minimal threshold for social niceties" (Roter & Hall, 1992, p. 91). In both cases, small talk at the beginning of the visit can act to (1) assess patients' state of mind and general well-being; and (2) create a more relaxed atmosphere in which to transition to the more transactional aspects of the visit (Coupland et al., 1994), both of which are important components in creating a positive provider–patient relationship as well as a way of treating the patient holistically rather than simply attending to the biomedical aspects of their patienthood.

3.3 *You Exercise Every Day?*

Small talk does not only occur at the 'edges' of visits but may also arise in the middle of the medical visit. This third excerpt comes from a visit between Karen and Mr. Eggers and occurs during the transition to the physical exam phase of the visit. At this point, the NP and patient both physically move from the desk area of the office to the examination table. This example also illustrates Maynard and Hudak's "disattentiveness-in-simultaneity" (2008), in which small talk occurs at a transition point within the visit. This example of small talk falls more toward the 'work' end of the continuum, something akin to "work-related talk" (Holmes, 2000) in that the topic is relevant to the medical visit and many of the utterances could be considered medically focused. The important shift away from the medical frame occurs in line 8, when Karen inquires where Mr. Eggers exercises.

Excerpt 3

1. Karen: let me examine you
2. Mr. Eggers: I'm ## well I've cut back a little bit but I'm in the gym
3.   every day
4. Karen: oh you do you exercise every day
5. Mr. Eggers: yeah
6. Karen: excellent for how many minutes
7. Mr. Eggers: well about forty five minutes for the whole workout

8. Karen: good where do you go
9. Mr. Eggers: I go to the Bartlett civic center
10. Karen: oh nice
11. Mr. Eggers: where it costs me forty dollars a year
12. Karen: forty dollars a year that's excellent
13. Mr. Eggers: hhh yeah
14. Karen: good for you cause-
15. Mr. Eggers: and then you know in the summer time I ###
16. Karen: yeah but the more you exercise the better you'll feel
17. all the way around in so many different aspects
18. Mr. Eggers: well its like I go in and I do six miles on the stationary bike
19. and then in the summer I'll do another ten twelve on my
20. own bike hhhhh
21. Karen: oh yeah that's excellent good good good

This exchange exemplifies what Hudak and Maynard (2011) refer to as "co-topical" small talk, or talk which represents a departure from the medical tasks at hand but is still relevant to the medical visit. In fact, in this exchange, it is difficult to determine if it is, in fact, even small talk. I argue that it is for two important reasons. First, it is not immediately relevant to the current task of the examination, which Karen announces in line 1. Instead, the patient, Mr. Eggers, initiates this topic unprompted, with no mention of exercise prior to this exchange. Second, Karen's inquiry as to where Mr. Eggers exercises is purely relational, suggesting a relational rather than a medical frame, and does not contribute to her knowledge about the type of exercise he does, how often, or for how long he exercises, all of which could be considered medically relevant. Karen's questions in line 4 ("do you exercise every day") and line 6 ("for how many minutes") could both be seen as performing a dual function of attending to relational as well as transactional goals and, in that way, could be an overlapping of the medical and relational frames. However, the question in line 8 is a departure from this and seems to be doing relational work only, both allowing Mr. Eggers to continue with this topic that he introduced and allowing him to share more of his personal life with her. He does, in fact, continue to share more about his experience at this gym when he tells her how much it costs him (line 11), an additional detail that does not provide any medical insight and can be argued as not directly relevant to the transactional goals of the medical visit. Karen's turn in line 14 is cut off by Mr. Eggers' sharing more information about his exercise routine. In this turn, it is unclear what Karen's intended utterance was. The use of "cause" (e.g. 'because') suggests a causal relation to the prior utterance regarding cost; however, she could also be responding to the exchange as a whole, providing an evaluation of his exercise habits in general, which is what she does in lines 16–17 before shifting topics altogether. In this way, there is a blurring between the relational and medical frames during this exchange.

In this excerpt, Karen and Mr. Eggers engage in small talk that is, for the most part, relevant to the medical visit, as it focuses on Mr. Eggers' exercise routine. There are elements that seem to be both relational as well as transactional, particularly the information that Mr. Eggers shares about how frequently he exercises (lines 3 and 7) and the type of exercise he does (lines 18–20). There are also elements which are beyond the scope of the medical visit, namely where Mr. Eggers goes to exercise and how much he pays for his membership. The departure into these topics suggest that Mr. Eggers in interacting within a relational frame, albeit one that is still medically relevant, suggesting an overlap, or blurring of these frames, which is likely common in the case where a provider and patient have already an existing professional relationship.[1]

3.4 Don't Go to the Grocery Store

This last excerpt is taken from Defibaugh (in press), in which I argue that small talk at the closings of medical visits allows providers to create a continuity of care (West, 2006) across visits, essentially laying the groundwork for the following visits. In this exchange, the patient, Mr. Quinn, is accompanied by his wife, Mrs. Quinn. This is the first visit between Sarah and the Quinns and, similar to many of the visits in the VA clinic, is an annual check-up for Mr. Quinn. Most of the exchange takes place between Mrs. Quinn and Sarah. This is also true for the bulk of the visit in which Mrs. Quinn often acts as a voice for Mr. Quinn, who is quite a bit older than his wife and has difficulty hearing. Unlike the previous example, the topic is completely unrelated to the medical visit or the patient's health. This exchange reflects a purely relational frame and seemingly performs an exclusively social function in which the NP seeks to create a positive relationship between herself, the patient and his wife. It occurs at the end of the visit, as Sarah is escorting the Quinns out of the examination room.

Excerpt 4

```
 1. Sarah:       okay:::.all right so you have a wonderful
 2.              Thanksgiving,=
 3. Mrs. Quinn:              =you [too
 4. Mr. Quinn:                    [hey you too
 5. Sarah:       you take her out (.) fer lunch
 6. Mrs. Quinn: ↑ today?
 7. Sarah:       [yeah
 8. Mrs. Quinn: [no he's going [to exercise
 9. Mr. Quinn:                 [it's time for her to take me out hhhh
10. Sarah:       hhhh although don't go to the grocery store (.) I
11.              went yesterday I thought I was going to die hhhh
12. Mrs. Quinn: OH MY GOSH I was there last weekend and it was
13.              so crowded=
14. Sarah:                  =it was [a:::wful
15. Mrs. Quinn:                     [I know::
16. Sarah:       I had to park my cart (.) on the side [of the (.)
17. Mrs. Quinn:                                        [hhhh
18. Sarah:       and the end and then walk down the aisle to get
19.              what I wanted it [was aw::ful=
20. Mr. Quinn:                   [yeah
21. Mrs. Quinn:                            = and nobody stole
22.              your cart? hhhh
23. Sarah:       no hhh (1.0) so [I told my husband 'I hope we
24. Mrs. Quinn:                  [it's terrible
25. Sarah:       don't need to go back [it's the worst
26. Mrs. Quinn:                        [my daughter's cooking but
27.              I'm I already got the sweet potatoes I'm gonna
28.              make [them
29. Sarah:            [hhhh
30. Mrs. Quinn: and I'mna make up the pies tomorrow I >already
31.              got it all<
32.              so (.) no: don't have to go to the store no more
33. Sarah:       I know all [right well thank you so much I'll
34. Mrs. Quinn:             [it's terrible
35. Sarah:       show you a shortcut if you don't have to go
36.              anywhere else
```

In line 1, Sarah initiates a closing sequence, signaling a transition from the previous topic to the close of the visit, marked with the use of "okay" and "all right." She wishes them a "wonderful Thanksgiving" (lines 1–2), which both Mr. and Mrs. Quinn recognize as a closing and respond accordingly. The visit could easily end here as Sarah could then "show (them) a shortcut" as she eventually does in line 35; however, she makes another closing move, telling Mr. Quinn to take his wife to lunch (line 5). Similar to the use of humor in excerpt 4, Sarah uses humor here to construct rapport with the Quinns. As noted in Defibaugh (in press), this is likely in reference to an earlier exchange in which Mr. Quinn jokingly referred to his wife as his secretary. By suggesting that Mr. Quinn should take his wife to lunch, she acknowledges that earlier exchange, constructing a kind of inside joke between the three of them. Mr. Quinn continues this joking rapport by suggesting that it is his wife's turn to take him out (line 9), which both he and Sarah respond to with brief laughter. Sarah then makes an additional relational move, extending the small talk exchange by introducing a new topic of grocery shopping in the days before Thanksgiving. She shares her recent experience (lines 10–11, 14, 16, 18–19), which Mrs. Quinn aligns with by sharing her own experience (12–13) as well as affective minimal responses ("I know" line 15, "it's terrible" line 24) and even attempts to contribute to Sarah's story ("and nobody stole your cart" 21–22), adding a potentially comical and frustrating detail. She also shares her Thanksgiving plans (lines 26–31), illustrating her engagement in this topic.

In this exchange, Sarah constructs a purely relational frame in which she shares her own experience with the patient and his wife, much like Ragan (2000) describes. However, in Ragan's (2000) example of the provider sharing personal experiences, these are still within a medical frame as the topic is based on the provider's experience with certain medications. In this exchange, the experience that Sarah shares is not related to her experience with medical care or medicine, but is purely relational. It cannot be said that her choice to share this has any effect on the transactional goals of the visit per se. Instead, the relational talk allows the two women to engage within a relational frame and bond over their negative experiences of recent grocery store visits, constructing a relationship that goes beyond their provider and patient identities, or in this case provider and patient's family member.[2] In Defibaugh (in press), I argue that by creating a positive relationship, Sarah is laying the groundwork for future visits, contributing to a continuity of care for the Quinns.

4   Conclusion

Much like the linguistic features discussed in other chapters, small talk performs multiple functions in terms of the enactment of professional competency. Small talk allows providers and patients to move beyond their institutionally defined roles and interact, albeit briefly, as equals. The NPs are able to access the patients' lifeworld (Mishler, 1984) by engaging in relational talk, which allows for topics such as exercise/gym memberships and shopping experiences, some of which may be medically relevant and some of which simply create a personal connection and rapport that is unrelated to the medical tasks at hand. NPs are more able to treat patients from a holistic perspective than focusing simply on their medical conditions when they are able to learn more about their daily life and personalities. Similarly, small talk may provide insights into health-related information and behavior that would not have arisen otherwise, as is the case with the discussion of Mr. Eggers' exercise routine. Finally, as discussed in Chap. 1, when patients feel as though their provider cares about them, they are more likely to adhere to medical treatment (Hayes, 2007). Small talk is a way for NPs to show interest and concern for patients beyond their immediate medical condition and their institutionally defined roles, a move that has the potential to positively influence health outcomes.

Moreover, as the examples illustrate, the line between what is work talk and what is small talk often gets blurred in medical visits. In initial exchanges, questions such as 'how are you' are primarily taken up by patients within the relational frame, evidenced by the fact that responses are often formulaic, routinized responses to greetings. These relational frames at the beginning of the visit are often minimally engaged in by both providers and patients as they quickly switch to more medically focused talk. Co-topical small talk, such as that discussed in excerpt 3 between Karen and Mr. Eggers, seems to perform both relational and transactional work, skirting the line between the relational and the medical frame. Talk such as this is difficult to neatly place into one of two categories, supporting Holmes' (2000) continuum model and Koester's (2010) multidimensional categories of workplace discourse.

Finally, most of the small talk exchanges are all relatively short, taking very little time away from the transactional work of the visit. Because of the benefits they can have on the provider–patient relationship, the use of small talk in short segments such as these likely contribute more to the visit than they actually detract from it, fitting what Roter and Hall refer to as the "minimum threshold for social niceties" (1992, p. 91). However, even longer small talk exchanges, when they occur at the end of the visit do not necessarily detract from the work talk, but enhance it by creating an atmosphere of "*genuine*, personal involvement and concern" (Coupland et al., 1994, p. 102).

Notes

1. The fact that Mr. Griffin so easily jokes with Karen and, even more significantly, that he brings her a gift, also reflects the current relationship between them.
2. Although the topic is, once again, based around the Thanksgiving holiday, the work that Sarah is doing is not atypical in medical visits. The holiday likely makes it easier to initiate small talk since there is a shared topic readily at hand; however, Sarah's first comment about Mr. Quinn taking his wife to lunch could have occurred at any time of the year and highlights her shift to a relational frame at the closing of the visit and her willingness to engage in non-work-related talk.

References

Coupland, J. (2000). Introduction: Sociolinguistic perspectives on small talk. In J. Coupland (Ed.), *Small talk* (pp. 1–26). London: Pearson.
Coupland, J., Robinson, J., & Coupland, N. (1994). Frame negotiation in doctor-elderly patient consultations. *Discourse & Communication, 5*(1), 89–124.
Defibaugh, S. (in press). Small talk as work talk: Enacting the patient-centered approach in nurse-practitioner- patient visits. *Communication and Medicine.*
Fraser, B. (1988). Types of English discourse markers. *Acta Linguistica Hungarica, 38*(1–4), 19–33.
Hayes, E. (2007). Nurse practitioners and managed care: Patient satisfaction and intention to adhere to nurse practitioner plan of care. *Journal of the American Academy of Nurse Practitioners, 19*, 418–426.
Holmes, J. (2000). Doing collegiality and keeping control at work: Small talk in government departments. In J. Coupland (Ed.), *Small talk* (pp. 27–31). London: Pearson.
Hudak, P., & Maynard, P. (2011). An interactional approach to conceptualising small talk in medical interactions. *Sociology of Health & Illness, 33*(4), 634–653.
Koester, A. (2010). *Workplace discourse.* London: Continuum.
Malinowski, B. (2006). On phatic communion. In N. Coupland & A. Jaworksi (Eds.), *The discourse reader* (2nd ed., pp. 296–298). New York: Routledge. (Original work published 1923).
Maynard, D., & Hudak, P. (2008). Small talk, high stakes: Interactional disattentiveness in the context of prosocial doctor-patient interaction. *Language in Society, 37*, 661–688.
McCarthy, M. (2000). Captive audiences: Small talk and close contact service encounters. In J. Coupland (Ed.), *Small talk* (pp. 84–109).

Mishler, E. (1984). *The discourse of medicine: Dialectics of medical interviews.* Norwood, NJ: Ablex.

Ragan, S. L. (2000). Sociable talk in women's health care contexts: Two forms of non-medical talk. In J. Coupland (Ed.), *Small talk* (pp. 269–287). London: Pearson.

Roter, D., & Hall, J. (1992/2006). *Doctors talking with patients/patients talking with doctors: Improving communication in medical visits* (2nd ed.). Westport, CT: Praeger.

Tannen, D. (1993). What's in a frame? Surface evidence for underlying expectations. In D. Tannen (Ed.), *Frame analysis* (pp. 14–56).

West, C. (2006). Coordinating care in primary care visits: Producing continuity of care. In J. Heritage & D. Maynard (Eds.), *Communication in medical care: Interaction between primary care physicians and patients* (pp. 379–415). Cambridge: Cambridge University Press.

Zimmerman, D. (1992). The interactional organization of calls for emergency assistance. In P. Drew & J. Heritage (Eds.), *Talk at work* (pp. 418–469).

CHAPTER 6

Conclusion

Abstract The enactment of professional competency is, of course, field dependent. In the case of medical care, nurse practitioners engage in a range of linguistic practices that require both technical and communication-based skills. Drawing on prior research of what effective communication looks like, this chapter brings together the four analysis chapters as well as the prior literature presented in the introduction, suggesting how linguistic analysis can add to our understanding of effective health communication. Although specific correlations cannot be made, it is possible to see how the patterns of talk align, to varying extents, with the prior research from the field of health communication, highlighting how the enactment of competency is accomplished through linguistic practices. The chapter concludes with suggestions for future avenues of research.

Keywords Health communication • Interactional practices • Medical discourse • Nurse practitioners • Professional competency

1 INTRODUCTION

This final chapter brings together the arguments presented in each of the prior chapters and ties these back to the concept of professional competence. First, I return to the main goals of the book, as set out in the preface

© The Author(s) 2018
S. Defibaugh, *Nurse Practitioners and the Performance of Professional Competency*, Communicating in Professions and Organizations, https://doi.org/10.1007/978-3-319-68354-6_6

and the introductory chapter, noting how the analysis of specific linguistic features may be associated with particular roles that nurse practitioners (NPs) play in their enactment of the patient-centered approach and how this approach has been associated with the core competencies defined by medical boards and identified in the research as entailing best practices in health care delivery. I provide a few caveats for the reader in terms of the claims that this book makes as well as a brief discussion of areas for future research.

2 Bringing It All Together

My primary goal in writing this book was to provide a kind of documentation of the interactional work that NPs engage in and to tie this to the large body of health communication research. As noted in the preface and introduction, a great deal of work has been done on medical discourse with doctors, and a great deal of health communication and evidence-based research has been done on NPs, but up until this point, an effort at connecting these two disciplines has not been attempted. By examining the interactions from the perspective of professional competency, my aim was to do just that. Drawing on what we know about professional competency and successful health outcomes, the research is clear that NPs perform equally and even better than other providers serving in similar roles. This is based on the two measures of patient satisfaction and improved health outcomes (see Chap. 1 for a full discussion). In the prior chapters, I have attempted to tie the linguistic features of NPs' interactional work to the concept of the patient-centered approach, which has been defined by numerous researchers, all of which include similar concepts. The key concepts in these definitions include a focus on building partnerships, enhancing the provider–patient relationship, encouraging shared decision making and negotiation of treatment, and engaging in health education. As outlined in Chap. 1, many of the features of patient-centered care align with the core competencies of medical boards including the National Organization for Nurse Practitioner Faculties (NONPF), the Accreditation Council for Graduate Medical Education (ACGME), and the American Board of Medical Specialties (ABMS), indicating a consensus across the medical community of the value of patient-centeredness. Throughout the book I have drawn connections between the features of patient-centered care with a number of specific linguistic practices. In the following paragraphs, I make these connections more explicitly.

The construction of provider–patient relationships has primarily been addressed in Chaps. 4 and 5 with their focus on indirectness and small talk, respectively. Indirectness creates a sense of optionality, lessening the sense of power between the NP and the patient, giving the impression of a more equitable relationship. Small talk constructs a relationship based not on the institutional roles of provider and patient but instead offers the opportunity for individuals to relate to one another on a more personal level by engaging in relational frames of talk.

The emphasis on patient education was the focus of Chap. 3. In this chapter, I primarily addressed how NPs share their expert knowledge with patients, adapting it to individual needs and making information relatable and easy to comprehend. Although not the focus of Chap. 4, educating patients is also part of advice-giving, and is often the indirect mechanism for offering advice and criticizing past behavior. For example, explanations of how to manage diabetes and the need to take all medications that are prescribed, and for that matter, not taking a medication that is no longer being prescribed, are ways of giving medical directives through education and information sharing.

Decision making and negotiation of treatment were not specifically addressed in any of the chapters but can be tied into the discussion of indirectness as well, specifically in how medical directives are presented with a sense of optionality. As I have argued, indirectness gives the impression of optionality to medical directives, making decisions seem to be open for discussion rather than simply dictated. Although the medical setting and care discussed in this book is quite different from the genetic counseling sessions described by Benkendorf et al. (2001), NPs do seem to draw on similar indirect means when giving medical directives, suggesting an overlap between nondirective medical care, the use of indirectness, and NPs' style in advice-giving. In post visit interviews, both Julie, working in the cardiac clinic, and Sarah, working in the outpatient clinic, described their role as a "guide" or "facilitator," explaining that their role is to provide information to patients and allow them to make their own decisions. In this way, the focus on education and the use of indirect speech may both be correlated with the patient-centered concept of shared decision making. Patient education provides patients with the knowledge and tools they need to make informed decisions; indirectness creates optionality in medical directives, leaving the choice of whether to follow the medical advice in the hands of the patient.

The one chapter that cannot be correlated with patient-centered care, is Chap. 2, which addresses organizational responsibilities. Although patient-centeredness is clearly an important part of what it means to be a competent medical provider, this book and its presentation of competency would be incomplete if it did not consider organizational factors that influence talk and that are part of what it means to be a health care provider. In Chap. 2, I highlight the ways that NPs balance their responsibility to their patients and their responsibility to their organizations as well as the ways in which these may overlap. Competency is multifaceted; part of what health care providers must do is work with colleagues on patient care and follow the guidelines provided by them. Prior research has noted that providers often control the talk of the visits by asking questions, including limiting these to yes/no questions and by holding the floor for extended periods of time (Atkinson, 1982; Heritage & Clayman, 2010; Roter & Hall, 1992). This has traditionally been understood as a reflection of the older, provider-centered model of care. As I hope I have shown throughout this book, NPs are engaging in patient-centered care, and yet, this feature of controlling the talk through the checklist is still present. The reason for this is likely that it is an inherent aspect of medical care and one that is reinforced by organizational requirements. NPs can engage in patient-centered care and still control the talk to some extent; these concepts are not necessarily in opposition to one another but simply reflect different aspects of a provider's professional competency.

3 A Constellation of Linguistic Resources

An important point to note in the closing of this book is that the linguistic features described throughout should not be taken in isolation. Instead, I ask that the reader view these as a constellation of linguistic resources that NPs draw upon in their interactions with patients. That is, it is not enough to say that engaging in small talk, in itself, creates a positive rapport with patients or should be interpreted as best practices. Instead, as I have pointed out, small talk in short segments can have the effect of lowering social distance, which can create a positive provider–patient relationship. This does not mean that small talk should be the bulk of the medical visit or that it alone is a display of professional competency. The engagement of small talk is simply one part of how NPs create rapport with patients, and creating rapport is just one aspect of what it means to be a competent medical provider. Likewise, providing education is clearly an important part of medical care, but it is not the only thing that an NP does that likely contributes to high satisfaction and positive health outcomes. Viewing the linguistic features as a set of practices illustrates the multiplicity of roles that NPs enact, which require them to balance organizational, transactional, and relational work within any given visit. Although it would be imprudent to make the claim based on the data presented herein, it is my belief that it is the balance of these various aspects of professional competency that makes NPs successful rather than any individual part.

It is also important to note that (1) the ways in which these competencies get enacted will vary by provider, (2) not all visits will have the same balance of the linguistic features described in this book, and (3) not all NPs will enact all aspects of their professional competency in each visit. The first point should already be obvious as each chapter presents multiple extracts that can be understood within the same larger framework, but illustrate variation in form. For example, in Chap. 3, I note the ways that patient education is accomplished and how different NPs may use different approaches to share knowledge with patients. Laura, for instance, is the only NP who translates the lipid panel into food choices. Although not included in the chapter, Julie provides statistics to patients on the fatality of influenza as a way to help the patient make an informed decision about getting the flu vaccine. Similarly, all NPs employ indirectness in some ways. June uses voicing of others often (Defibaugh, 2014a), and although others do not do this, they use other forms of indirect speech. Individual variation is a reflection both of NPs meeting various patients' needs as well as a reflection of their individual style.

To address the second point, it is important to note that individual visits vary in terms of the balancing of various competencies or the ways in which certain aspects of patient-centered care become foregrounded or backgrounded in the visit. The example of the visit between June and Ms. Piper is a clear example of how patient education may be primary in the interaction, with other interactional features being less prominent. In other visits, June spends the bulk of her time working on coordinating care with patients and imparts very little education. In some of the outpatient VA clinic visits, the NPs' job seems to be mainly to verify the patient's health information in order to update the electronic medical records and renew prescriptions. Patients' needs vary, and the care they receive will vary as well, leading to certain aspects of the NPs' professional competency to be highlighted in a greater way than others in any given interaction.

The final point, although quite similar but worthy of a brief discussion in its own right, is that not all NPs will enact all aspects of their professional competency in each visit. This variation can partly be attributed to the settings in which the NPs practice and the goals of each visit. June, for example, engages in much less small talk than her counterparts working in outpatient settings. The reason for this may be the fact that she has an opportunity to get to know patients and build rapport with them over the course of multiple visits within any given hospitalization rather than seeing them sporadically over the course of a year, which is typical for outpatient care. It is also likely a reflection of my data collection methods; with June, I observed one visit with each patient, but this could have been an initial visit or a follow-up visit. To be clear, June does engage in small talk with patients occasionally. In Defibaugh (2014b), I discuss an exchange between Ms. Piper and June in which they discuss Ms. Piper's occupation, delving into topics that are not medically relevant in the same way that the exchange between Karen and Mr. Griffin reveals aspects of his non-patient identity.

One way to view these differences is again to return to the notion of the patient-centered approach. One of the defining features is addressing individual patient needs and treating them holistically rather than simply as human embodiments of disease or illness. In the case of Ms. Piper, she needs reassurance about her new diagnosis and focused information that addresses her immediate needs. Mr. Stevens, another patient of June's (discussed in Chap. 3), already has a great deal of knowledge about diabetes, and instead, needs further support to continue making the improvements he has been working toward. In an outpatient setting, patients' needs are often quite different. Again, not discussed in great detail in this book, the example of small talk between Sarah and the Quinns is likely an example of how the NP adapts her talk to the needs of the patient. In this instance, there had been a strain in the relationship between the Quinns and the VA that Sarah is attempting to repair (see Defibaugh, in press), which could explain why she engages in a lengthy small talk exchange with them, but not with all patients. The similarities in interactional norms suggests that their training as NPs leads them to engage in particular practices, but the variation across visits can be understood as individual stylistic choices on the part of the NP as well as adapting to individual patients' needs.

CONCLUSION 127

4 FUTURE DIRECTIONS

I close this chapter by discussing some of the limitations of this book and the ways in which the research can be expanded upon to better address larger questions of how specific linguistic practices can be understood alongside the findings of health communication researchers. First, the approach to the data that I took in this book differs from much of the prior work on medical discourse in that I organized the analytic chapters around a set of features that can roughly be associated with different aspects of professional competency. Much of the prior discourse-based research on medical care has examined what happens during particular structural phases of the visit. What became clear for me, in the process of analyzing the data, was that these competencies, as I have referred to them, occur across different phases. Attending to the medical checklist, for instance, has been discussed in terms of the history-taking phase of the visit (Boyd & Heritage, 2006) but in the case of annual well-visit exams will often happen throughout the course of the visit, with deviations from this checklist also occurring throughout. Similarly, small talk is not simply relegated to openings but may occur at various points in the visit and even continue after the work of the visit is completed. Patient education also occurs at various points in a visit and, sometimes, may comprise the majority of the visit. Looking at the data from this perspective highlights how NPs are enacting multiple competencies at any given point in a visit. In a similar vein, Zayts and Schnurr (2014) approach the discourse of nurses in genetic counseling sessions as the performance of various roles. I could also argue that the competencies encompass particular roles or identities—for example, the role of educator or the role of organizational team member. Drawing further connection between the competencies, the roles or identities and the ways in which these may occur within and/or across the structural phases would be worth exploring in order to better understand both the phases of medical visits (and what roles may play a more prominent part, for instance) as well as why different roles may come to the forefront in a given visit or in a particular phase of the visit.

Additionally, I have utilized data from various sources that represent different settings rather than examining the practices of NPs in one particular setting. I believe this is a strength of the present analysis in that it reveals the patterns of talk that occur across different settings and, as I noted in the previous section, may also reveal ways in which the various settings reveal variability in the nature of the talk. There is still more to be done in this area. NPs practice in a wide variety of settings and research that explores the interactional practices in all of these settings can expand our understanding of their interactional practices. Furthermore, the regulations on NPs vary by state within the United States. If this remains the case, then these factors need to be taken into account and data in which different regulations are in place should be examined; the ways in which those regulations may influence an NP's practice should also be considered. Just as I have discussed how the organizational responsibilities influence the medical visit, constraints on a NPs' practice will also influence the talk. Although the NPs included in this book represent different work settings, there is still a limited number of NPs and a limited number of settings. This book is intended to present some of the features of NP–patient talk and to highlight the ways that NPs, through the use of particular linguistic practices interact with patients. However, future work may include larger number of providers working in different medical settings.

Moreover, the gender bias for NPs as a whole and for my data set is something that cannot be ignored. The NPs in this study, while fairly representative of the profession as a whole, are all female. It is quite possible that some of the linguistic practices discussed here are influenced by the NPs' gender; the only way to more accurately address this is to include male NPs in future research. This would also need to be taken into consideration if one were interested in a comparison with other provider types in which there is greater gender variation.

5 Conclusion

In this book, I have shown how the linguistic practices of NPs may reflect their patient-centered approach and how this approach is correlated with the concept of professional competency. Although I cannot correlate these practices with the positive health outcomes and high patient satisfaction ratings that NPs are often associated with, a fine-grained analysis does contribute to our understanding, providing additional data that can be used to triangulate results and offer potential explanations for them. By incorporating the work of health communication scholars and the core competencies of various medical accreditation boards, I hope that this book has made headway in crossing disciplinary boundaries and in advancing our understanding of discursive practices in medical settings.

References

Atkinson, J. M. (1982). Understanding formality: The categorization and production of 'formal interaction'. *British Journal of Sociology, 33*(1), 86–117.

Benkendorf, J. L., Prince, M. B., Rose, M. A., De Fina, A., & Hamilton, H. E. (2001). Does indirect speech promote nondirective genetic counseling? Results of a sociolinguistic investigation. *American Journal of Medical Genetics, 106*, 199–207.

Boyd, E., & Heritage, J. (2006). Taking the history: Questioning during comprehensive history-taking. In J. Heritage & D. W. Maynard (Eds.), *Communication in medicine* (pp. 151–184). Cambridge: Cambridge University Press.

Defibaugh, S. (2014a). Management of health or management of face: Indirectness in nurse practitioner-patient interactions. *Journal of Pragmatics, 67*, 61–71.

Defibaugh, S. (2014b). Solidarity and alignment in nurse practitioner/patient interactions. *Discourse & Communication, 8*(3), 260–277.

Defibaugh, S. (in press). Small talk as work talk: Enacting the patient-centered approach in nurse-practitioner- patient visits. *Communication and Medicine*.

Heritage, J., & Clayman, S. (2010). *Talk in action: Interactions, identities, and institutions*. Oxford: Wiley-Blackwell.

Roter, D., & Hall, J. (1992/2006). *Doctors talking with patients/patients talking with doctors: Improving communication in medical visits* (2nd ed.). Westport, CT: Praeger.

Zayts, O., & Schnurr, S. (2014). More than 'information provider' and 'counselor': Constructing and negotiating roles and identities of nurses in genetic counseling sessions. *Journal of SocioLinguistics, 18*(3), 345–369.

Erratum to: Nurse Practitioners and the Performance of Professional Competency: Accomplishing Patient-centered Care

Staci Defibaugh

Erratum to:
S. Defibaugh, *Nurse Practitioners and the Performance of Professional Competency: Accomplishing Patient-centered Care*, Communicating in Professions and Organizations,
https://doi.org/10.1007/978-3-319-68354-6

An error in the production process led to the publication of this book prematurely, before the incorporation of some corrections. Extracts and their in-text references have been updated and the corrected version has been approved by the author.

The updated online version of this book can be found at
https://doi.org/10.1007/978-3-319-68354-6

© The Author(s) 2018
S. Defibaugh, *Nurse Practitioners and the Performance of Professional Competency*, Communicating in Professions and Organizations,
https://doi.org/10.1007/978-3-319-68354-6_7

Index[1]

A
Adherence, 10, 11, 40
Advice, 9, 19, 83–98, 106, 107, 123
Asymmetrical, 37, 59, 74
Asymmetry, vii, 5, 59, 60, 65, 112

B
Back region, 29
Backstage, 18, 19, 28
 See also Back region
Bivalent, 81, 87, 97

C
Checklist, 32, 34–41, 49, 124, 127
Communication, vii, viii, 6, 9–14, 28, 29, 46, 48, 54, 60, 107, 122, 127, 128

Competencies, viii, 6, 9–14, 19, 20, 28–32, 34, 37, 41, 44, 46, 48, 49, 54, 80, 98, 101, 105, 117, 121, 122, 124–128
Coordinating care, 28, 30–34, 42–48, 125
Coordination, 4, 19, 30, 33
Criticism, 19, 84, 97
Critiques, 80, 83, 84, 97

D
Directives, 19, 20, 70, 79, 123
Doctors, 5, 9, 11, 17, 32, 35, 103, 105

E
Education, 6, 8, 9, 16, 19, 33, 42, 44, 54–75, 123–125, 127

---

[1]Note: Page numbers followed by "n" refers to notes.

Electronic medical records (EMRs), 19, 28, 30–32, 34, 40, 41, 46, 49, 50n1, 125
Epistemic access, 57, 58, 60, 63, 66–70, 72–74
Epistemic primacy, 19, 57, 58, 71–73
Epistemic responsibility, 54

F
Frames, 7, 39, 54, 63, 91, 97, 106–115, 117, 118, 119n2
Front region, 29, 35, 42, 48
Frontstage, 19, 28–49
  See also Front region

H
Health care, 2–4, 6–14, 21n1, 32, 48, 49, 54, 55, 73, 75, 107, 124
Health outcomes, 6, 10–12, 14, 55, 75, 102, 118, 122, 125, 128
Hedges, 58, 82, 84, 95
Hedging, 58, 85, 91, 95, 97

I
Implicature, 81, 82, 85, 92
Indirect, 5, 19, 79–98, 103, 123, 125
Indirectness, 9, 19, 80–85, 87, 92, 94, 95, 97, 98, 123, 125
Information sharing, 19, 54, 64, 93, 123
Inpatient, viii, 3, 14, 16, 19, 28, 30, 33, 34, 42, 67, 74, 85
Instrumental, 102, 103, 105

Interactional, vii, viii, 5, 6, 14, 18, 30, 31, 37, 57–59, 74, 82, 88, 103, 105, 107, 122, 125, 126, 128
Interpersonal, 10, 13, 14, 83, 84, 102, 106

K
Knowledge, vii, 9, 19, 33, 41, 43, 49, 54–65, 67, 68, 71–75, 91, 92, 114, 123, 125, 126
Knowledge sharing, 54–57, 59, 61, 73, 75, 92

M
MDs, see Medical doctors
Medical care, vii, viii, 6, 9, 13, 19, 31, 33, 83, 107, 117, 123–125, 127
Medical doctors (MDs), vii, viii, 2–9, 13, 31, 33
Mitigate, 20, 65, 82–84, 88, 91
Mitigation, 58, 82–85, 88, 91, 97

N
NP-patient, viii, 5, 128

O
Off record, 80, 82, 83, 85, 92, 94, 97, 98
On record, 80, 82, 83, 86, 88, 92, 94–96
Organization, viii, 18–20, 28, 32, 33, 37, 40, 41, 44, 48, 124
Organizational, viii, 9, 18, 19, 28, 124, 125, 127, 128
Outcomes, viii, 6, 10, 11, 55, 75, 118, 122, 125, 128

Outpatient, viii, 3, 4, 15, 19, 28, 30, 32, 34, 35, 49, 61, 69, 74, 108, 109, 123, 125, 126

P
PAs, *see* Physician assistants
Patient-centered, 4, 8, 12, 13, 20, 54, 55, 65, 84, 98, 107, 109, 123–126, 128
Patient satisfaction, viii, 6–11, 122, 128
Physician assistants (PAs), vii, 4–7
Physicians, 3, 4, 6, 9, 12, 31, 32, 54, 56, 94, 107
Practitioner-patient, 4–6
Provider-patient, 2, 8, 12, 20, 28–30, 44, 56, 59, 80, 85, 98, 102, 107, 108, 113, 118, 124

R
Rapport, 9, 11, 20, 64, 107, 109, 110, 112, 117, 118, 124, 126

Relational, 83, 85, 98, 102, 104, 105, 107–115, 117, 118, 125
Roles, vii, 2–4, 7, 9, 10, 12, 15, 16, 18, 20, 28, 30–34, 37, 42–45, 54, 57–59, 74, 75, 91, 93, 94, 105, 107, 112, 117, 118, 122, 123, 125, 127

S
Small talk, 9, 20, 101–118, 124, 126, 127

T
Transactional, 18, 20, 102–115, 117, 118, 125

V
Voices, 96

The manufacturer's authorised representative in the EU is Springer Nature Customer Service Centre GmbH, Europaplatz 3, 69115 Heidelberg, Germany. If you have any concerns regarding our products, please contact ProductSafety@springernature.com

Printed and bound by CPI Group (UK) Ltd, Croydon, CR0 4YY
25/03/2026
02077952-0001